BMA

BMA

MEASUREMENT
IN
ULTRASOUND

MEASUREMENT
IN
ULTRASOUND

A practical handbook

2nd edition

Paul S. Sidhu BSc MBBS MRCP FRCR DTM&H
Consultant Radiologist
Department of Radiology
King's College Hospital
London, UK

Wui K. Chong MBBS MRCP FRCR
Associate Professor
University of North Carolina Hospital
Department of Radiology
Chapel Hill
North Carolina, USA

Keshthra Satchithananda BDS, FDSRCS, MBBS, FRCS, FRCR, CON
Consultant Radiologist
Department of Radiology
King's College Hospital
London, UK

CRC Press
Taylor & Francis Group
Boca Raton London New York

CRC Press is an imprint of the
Taylor & Francis Group, an **informa** business

CRC Press
Taylor & Francis Group
6000 Broken Sound Parkway NW, Suite 300
Boca Raton, FL 33487-2742

© 2016 by Taylor & Francis Group, LLC
CRC Press is an imprint of Taylor & Francis Group, an Informa business

No claim to original U.S. Government works

Printed and bound in India by Replika Press Pvt. Ltd.

Printed on acid-free paper
Version Date: 20151103

International Standard Book Number-13: 978-1-4822-3135-9 (Paperback)

This book contains information obtained from authentic and highly regarded sources. While all reasonable efforts have been made to publish reliable data and information, neither the author[s] nor the publisher can accept any legal responsibility or liability for any errors or omissions that may be made. The publishers wish to make clear that any views or opinions expressed in this book by individual editors, authors or contributors are personal to them and do not necessarily reflect the views/opinions of the publishers. The information or guidance contained in this book is intended for use by medical, scientific or health-care professionals and is provided strictly as a supplement to the medical or other professional's own judgement, their knowledge of the patient's medical history, relevant manufacturer's instructions and the appropriate best practice guidelines. Because of the rapid advances in medical science, any information or advice on dosages, procedures or diagnoses should be independently verified. The reader is strongly urged to consult the relevant national drug formulary and the drug companies' and device or material manufacturers' printed instructions, and their websites, before administering or utilizing any of the drugs, devices or materials mentioned in this book. This book does not indicate whether a particular treatment is appropriate or suitable for a particular individual. Ultimately it is the sole responsibility of the medical professional to make his or her own professional judgements, so as to advise and treat patients appropriately. The authors and publishers have also attempted to trace the copyright holders of all material reproduced in this publication and apologize to copyright holders if permission to publish in this form has not been obtained. If any copyright material has not been acknowledged please write and let us know so we may rectify in any future reprint.

Library of Congress Cataloging-in-Publication Data

Names: Sidhu, Paul S., author, editor. | Chong, Wui K., editor. |
Satchithananda, Keshthra, editor.
Title: Measurement in ultrasound / editors, Paul S. Sidhu, Wui K. Chong, and
Keshthra Satchithananda.
Description: Second edition. | Boca Raton : Taylor & Francis/CRC Press, 2016.
| Includes bibliographical references and index.
Identifiers: LCCN 2015040348 | ISBN 9781482231359 (alk. paper)
Subjects: | MESH: Ultrasonography--methods--Handbooks. | Reference
Values--Handbooks.
Classification: LCC RC78.7.U4 | NLM WN 39 | DDC 616.07/543--dc23
LC record available at http://lccn.loc.gov/2015040348

**Visit the Taylor & Francis Web site at
http://www.taylorandfrancis.com**

**and the CRC Press Web site at
http://www.crcpress.com**

CONTENTS

PEDIATRIC AND NEONATAL

EDITORS

P. S. Sidhu BSc, MBBS, MRCP, FRCR, DTM&H
Professor of Imaging Sciences
King's College London
Consultant Radiologist
Department of Clinical Radiology
King's College Hospital
Denmark Hill
London SE5 9RS
United Kingdom

W. K. Chong MBBS, MRCP, FRCR,
Associate Professor
University of North Carolina Hospital
Department of Radiology
2016 Old Clinic Bldg, CB#7510
Chapel Hill
North Carolina 27599-7510
United States of America

Keshthra Satchithananda BDS, FDSRCS, MBBS, FRCS, FRCR
Consultant Radiologist
Department of Radiology
King's College Hospital
Denmark Hill
London SE5 9RS
United Kingdom

CONTRIBUTING AUTHORS

Bhavna Batohi MBBS, FRCR
Department of Clinical Radiology
King's College Hospital
London, UK

Wui K. Chong MBBS, MRCP, FRCR
Department of Radiology
University of North Carolina Hospital
Chapel Hill, North Carolina, USA

Colin R. Deane PhD, MIPEM
Department of Medical Engineering and Physics
King's College Hospital
London, UK

Annamaria Deganello MD
Department of Radiology
King's College Hospital
London, UK

Induni Douglas MBBS, MD (RADIOLOGY)
Department of Radiology
National Hospital of Sri Lanka
Colombo, Sri Lanka

David Elias MBBS, MRCP, FRCR
Department of Radiology
Kings College Hospital
London, UK

Venus Hedayati MBBS, BSc, MRCP, FRCR
Department of Radiology
King's College Hospital
London, UK

Dean Y. Huang BMedSci, BMBS, MRCPCH, FRCR, EBIR
Department of Radiology
King's College Hospital
London, UK

Anu E. Obaro BSc, MBBS, FRCR
Department of Clinical Radiology
King's College Hospital
London, UK

Suzanne M. Ryan MRCPI, FRCR
Department of Radiology
King's College Hospital
London, UK

Keshthra Satchithananda BDS, FDSRCS, MBBS, FRCS, FRCR
Department of Radiology
King's College Hospital
London, UK

Maria E. K. Sellars MBChB, FRCR
Department of Radiology
King's College Hospital
London, UK

Paul S. Sidhu BSc, MBBS, MRCP, FRCR, DTM&H
Department of Radiology
King's College Hospital
London, UK

Anthony E. Swartz BS, RT(R), RDMS
WakeMed Physician Practices
Maternal-Fetal Medicine
Raleigh, North Carolina, USA

Adults

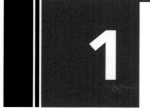

1

UPPER ABDOMINAL

Anu E. Obaro, Venus
Hedayati, Colin R. Deane,
Keshthra Satchithananda, and
Paul S. Sidhu

Liver size

PREPARATION
None.

POSITION
Supine, right anterior oblique to demonstrate the porta hepatis.

TRANSDUCER
2.0–6.0 MHz curvilinear transducer.

METHOD
Longitudinal views are taken in the midclavicular and midline positions, and measurements obtained. Anteroposterior diameters are also measured at the midpoint of the longitudinal diameters. All measurements are taken on deep inspiration.

APPEARANCE
Uniform pattern of medium-strength echoes.

MEASUREMENTS
There are significant variations in liver size due to gender, age, body mass index and weight.

Diameter	Female cm (mean $\pm$ SD)	Male cm (mean $\pm$ SD)
Midclavicular line (largest craniocaudal diameter)	14.9 $\pm$ 1.6	15.1 $\pm$ 1.5

Age (years)	Midclavicular line liver diameter cm (mean $\pm$ SD)
18–25	13.6 $\pm$ 1.5
26–35	13.7 $\pm$ 1.6
36–45	14.0 $\pm$ 1.6
46–55	14.2 $\pm$ 1.7
56–65	14.4 $\pm$ 1.8
$\geq$ 66	14.1 $\pm$ 2.0

In the transverse plane, the normal caudate lobe should be less than 2/3 of the size of the right lobe.

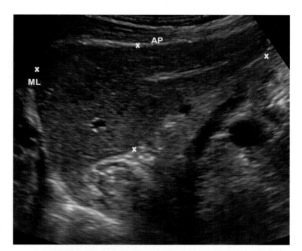

A midline longitudinal view through the left lobe of the liver, demonstrating the anteroposterior diameter (AP) and the midline longitudinal length (ML).

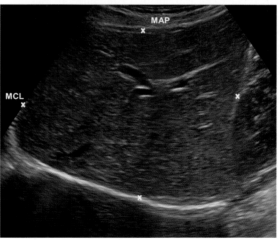

A midclavicular longitudinal view through the right lobe of the liver, with a midclavicular anteroposterior diameter (MAP) and a midclavicular longitudinal length (MCL).

FURTHER READING

Kratzer W, Fritz V, Mason RA, Haenle MM, Kaechele V. Factors affecting liver size: A sonographic survey of 2080 subjects. *J Ultrasound Med*. 2003; 22:1155–1161.

Patzak M, Porzner M, Oeztuerk S, Mason RA, Wilhelm M, Graeter T, Kratzer W, Haenle MM, Akinli AS. Assessment of liver size by ultrasonography. *J Clin Ultrasound*. 2014; 42:399–404.

Liver fibrosis assessment

PREPARATION
Patient should fast for 6–8 hours prior to the examination.

POSITION
Supine, right anterior oblique.

TRANSDUCER
2.0–6.0 MHz curvilinear transducer.

METHOD
Measurements are obtained from an intercostal view, to interrogate an area of the liver at least 2 cm deep to the liver capsule, away from major vessels. The right arm is raised above the head. The sample box is placed over the area selected, ideally in a perpendicular position, and a total of 10 measurements are obtained in brief suspended respiration, from the same area of liver. Segments 5 and 6 are normally interrogated; the left lobe of the liver should be avoided. Different ultrasound machines have different methods of obtaining readings and different display methods, and the readings are not transferable between machines. Transient elastography (TE) or "fibroscan" and acoustic radiation force impulse (ARFI) imaging are the most commonly used methods. A fibroscan does not produce an ultrasound image, and provides measurements in kilopascals (kPa).

APPEARANCE
The measurements can be expressed in velocity of shear wave (m/sec). The level of liver fibrosis is calculated and classified according to the METAVIR (F0–F4) or ISHAK (0–6) scoring system to ascertain normality, the degree of liver fibrosis, or the presence of cirrhosis. The most common diseases for which fibrosis will be assessed are Hepatitis C virus (HCV), Hepatitis B virus (HBV), and alcoholic liver disease.

MEASUREMENTS
Acoustic radiation force impulse (ARFI) imaging
(using a Siemens S2000, Mountain View, CA)

Healthy volunteers
1.07–1.19 m/s

HCV cutoff measurements for fibrosis (METAVIR SCORE)
   F ≥ 1 1.18–1.19 m/s
   F ≥ 2 1.21–1.34 m/s
   F ≥ 3 1.54–1.61 m/s
   F = 4 1.81–2.0 m/s

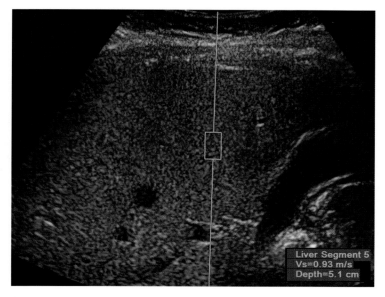

Liver Segment 5
Vs=0.93 m/s
Depth=5.1 cm

The "box" has been placed in the center of the right liver lobe and a measurement obtained for an ARFI measurement, estimated at 0.93 m/s.

FURTHER READING

Friedrich-Rust M, Nierhoff J, Lupsor M, Sporea I, Fierbinteanu-Braticevici C, Strobel D, Takahashi H, Yoneda M, Suda T, Zeuzem S, Herrmann E. Performance of Acoustic Radiation Force Impulse imaging for the staging of liver fibrosis: A pooled meta-analysis. *J Viral Hepat.* 2012; 19:e212–219.

Sporea I, Bota S, Săftoiu A, Şirli R, Gradinăru-Taşcău O, Popescu A, Lupşor Platon M, Fierbinteanu-Braticevici C, Gheonea DI, Săndulescu L, Badea R. Romanian national guidelines and practical recommendations on liver elastography. *Med Ultrason.* 2014; 6:123–138.

Biliary tree

PREPARATION
Patient should fast for 6–8 hours prior to the examination.

POSITION
Initially supine, then turn to the right anterior oblique or lateral decubitis positions to demonstrate the common duct.

TRANSDUCER
2.0–6.0 MHz curvilinear transducer.

METHOD
Patient is imaged from a subcostal position in the longitudinal plane or from an intercostal position. The common duct is measured at the point that passes anterior to the right portal vein, often with the hepatic artery seen in cross section between the duct and the vein. Intrahepatic ducts are measured at the level of the portal bifurcation. Color Doppler can be used to confirm the vascular and ductal anatomy. Measurements are taken from inner wall to inner wall and should be perpendicular to the course of the duct.

APPEARANCE
The extrahepatic bile duct may be divided into three segments: the hilar segment in front of the main portal vein, the suprapancreatic segment, and the intrapancreatic segment, which is ventral to the inferior vena cava (IVC) and passes through the pancreatic head. The maximal anteroposterior diameter of the extrahepatic bile duct is measured.

MEASUREMENTS
The extrahepatic duct may be measured at three locations: in the porta hepatis (proximal), in the most distal aspect of the head of the pancreas (distal), and midway between these measurements (middle). Average measurement for a normal adult common bile duct is 4 mm, though up to 6 mm is accepted as normal.

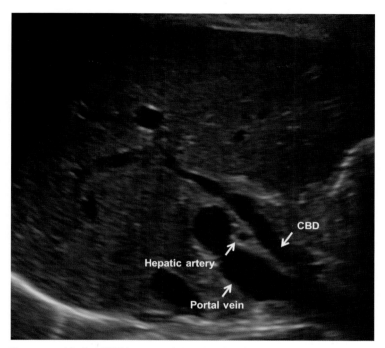

The common bile duct (CBD) is measured at a point where it passes anterior to the right portal vein, with the hepatic artery seen in cross section between the duct and the portal vein.

Location		Measurement mm (mean ± SD)
CBD	Proximal	2.9 ± 1.1
	Middle	3.5 ± 1.2
	Distal	3.5 ± 1.2
Intrahepatic duct	Right	1.9 ± 1.9
	Left	1.9 ± 1.1

In patients who have undergone a cholecystectomy, the common duct is significantly more distended by 3 months postoperative.

Location	Measurement preoperative mm (mean $\pm$ SD)	Measurement at 180 days mm (mean $\pm$ SD)
Proximal	2.27 $\pm$ 0.18	2.85 $\pm$ 0.20
Middle	3.49 $\pm$ 0.23	4.03 $\pm$ 0.25
Distal	4.31 $\pm$ 0.30	5.36 $\pm$ 0.33
Overall mean	3.32 $\pm$ 0.99	4.15 $\pm$ 1.26

There is an age-dependent change in the diameter of the common duct, and it can be up to 10 mm in the very elderly.

Common bile duct size variation with age

Age (years)	CBD diameter mm (mean $\pm$ SD)
20–30	2.7 $\pm$ 0.74
31–40	3.0 $\pm$ 0.81
41–50	3.5 $\pm$ 0.83
51–60	3.6 $\pm$ 0.81
71–80	4.3 $\pm$ 1.00
$\geq$ 81	5.0 $\pm$ 1.10

FURTHER READING

Bachar GN, Cohen M, Belenky A, Atar E, Gideon S. Effect of aging on the adult extrahepatic bile duct: A sonographic study. *J Ultrasound Med.* 2003; 22:879–882.

Matcuk GR, Grant EG, Ralls PW. Ultrasound measurements of the bile ducts and gallbladder: Normal ranges and effects of age, sex, cholecystectomy, and pathologic states. *Ultrasound Quarterly.* 2014; 30:41–48.

McArthur TA, Planz V, Fineberg NS, Tessler FN, Robbin ML, Lockhart ME. The common duct dilates after cholecystectomy and with advancing age: Reality or myth? *J Ultrasound Med.* 2013; 32:1385–1391.

Valkovic P, Miletic D, Zelic M, Brkljacic B. Dynamic changes in the common bile duct after laparoscopic cholecystectomy: A prospective longitudinal sonographic study. *Ultraschall Med.* 2011; 32:479–484.

Gallbladder and gallbladder wall

PREPARATION
Patient should fast for 6–8 hours prior to the examination.

POSITION
Initially supine, then a right anterior oblique position to ensure any small mobile stones are not missed.

TRANSDUCER
2.0–6.0 MHz curvilinear transducer.

METHOD
Longitudinal and transverse images are taken from a subcostal or an intercostal approach on deep inspiration in the supine and right anterior oblique positions.

APPEARANCE
On a longitudinal image the gallbladder appears as an echo-free pear-shaped structure. The gallbladder wall is smooth and is seen as a line of high reflectivity.

MEASUREMENTS
There is considerable variation in the size and shape of the gallbladder; however, certain reference values do exist.

Length (mm)	Width (mm)	Wall thickness mm (mean ± SD)
100 (range 80–120)	40–50	2.6 ± 1.6

FURTHER READING
Matcuk GR, Grant EG, Ralls PW. Ultrasound measurements of the bile ducts and gallbladder: Normal ranges and effects of age, sex, cholecystectomy, and pathologic states. *Ultrasound Quarterly*. 2014; 30:41–48.

Yarmenitis SD. Ultrasound of the gallbladder and the biliary tree. *Eur Radiol*. 2002; 12:270–282.

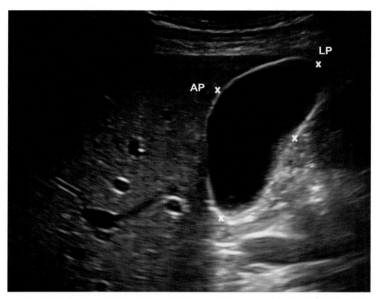

Longitudinal measurement (LP) of the gallbladder, and transverse diameter (AP) of the mid-aspect of the gallbladder.

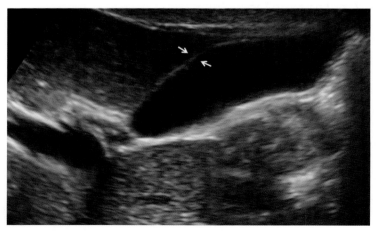

The thickness of the gallbladder wall is measured along the long axis of the ultrasound beam in an area where the gallbladder is contiguous with the liver.

Spleen

PREPARATION
None.

POSITION
Left upper abdomen in the mid-axillary line, then turn patient to left anterior oblique position as necessary to view the spleen.

TRANSDUCER
2.0–6.0 MHz curvilinear transducer.

METHOD
Splenic length measured during quiet breathing, obtained from a coronal plane that includes the hilum. The greatest longitudinal distance between the splenic dome and the tip (splenic length) is measured. Transverse, longitudinal and diagonal diameters are measured from the image showing maximum cross-sectional area in a coronal plane.

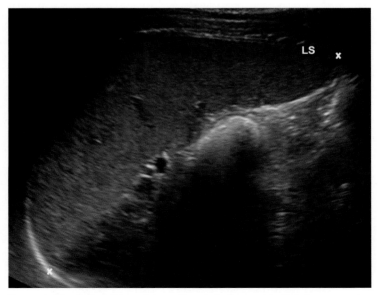

The greatest longitudinal distance between the splenic dome and the tip is the measured splenic length (LS).

APPEARANCE
The spleen is crescent shaped with a smooth convex diaphragmatic border and, often, a nodular concave medial border, which at the hilum contains the major splenic vessels and lymphatic channels.

The spleen should show a uniform homogeneous echo pattern, slightly more reflective than the liver, and should be considerably more reflective than the renal cortex.

An accessory spleen (10% multiple; 90% solitary) is found in up to 25% of the population, usually at the lower pole and most commonly up to 25 mm in diameter. An accessory spleen should be of a homogenous echo-texture to the spleen but can sometimes be difficult to differentiate from enlarged peri-splenic lymph nodes.

The tail of the pancreas may be seen adjacent to the splenic hilum.

MEASUREMENTS
Measurement of length: A measurement of length and diameter can be made in the oblique plane at the 10th and 11th intercostal space, through the splenic hilum (length ≤12 cm, diameter ≤7 cm).

The size of the spleen tends to increase with the subject's weight and height, but for the majority a size >13 cm length is considered abnormal. With increasing age there tends to be a reduction in the size of the spleen.

The volume and weight depend on the circulating blood volume. On average, the spleen is 10.9 ± 1.4 cm long, 4.0 ± 0.45 cm wide, 6.8 ± 0.71 cm in diameter, and weighs 150 to 200 g, in adult Caucasian patients.

Normal spleen lengths with age (in a Chinese population)

Age range in years	Male cm (mean ± SD)	Female cm (mean ± SD)
0–4	5.94 ± 1.18	5.77 ± 1.21
5–9	7.81 ± 1.28	7.48 ± 1.21
10–14	9.10 ± 1.41	8.76 ± 1.10
15–19	10.04 ± 1.29	8.61 ± 1.03
20–29	9.57 ± 1.05	9.08 ± 1.26

continued overleaf

Age range in years	Male cm (mean ± SD)	Female cm (mean ± SD)
30–39	9.52 ± 1.29	8.88 ± 1.28
40–49	9.38 ± 1.48	8.92 ± 1.54
50–59	8.83 ± 1.33	8.25 ± 1.39
60–69	8.99 ± 1.61	8.66 ± 1.50
70–79	8.60 ± 1.62	8.25 ± 1.54
80–89	7.90 ± 1.85	7.59 ± 1.53

Spleen size with sex, gender and race in collegiate athletes

	Height (m)	BMI (kg/m^2)	Length of spleen (cm)
Female	1.46	22.3	9.9
Male	1.84	25.9	11.3
African American	1.82	26.4	9.8
White	1.75	23.8	10.8

Measurement of area: View the spleen in the longitudinal axis, in deep inspiration. The interface between the lung and spleen serves as the transverse diameter, and the longitudinal diameter is measured from here to the splenic tip. The diagonal diameter is measured from this lateral spleen-lung interface to the medial spleen margin. The cross-sectional area is calculated as follows:

$$\frac{\text{Diagonal}}{\sqrt{(\text{Transverse}^2 + \text{Longitudinal}^2)/2}}$$

Normal	Diameter cm (mean ± SD)
Transverse diameter	5.5 ± 1.4
Longitudinal diameter	5.8 ± 1.8
Diagonal diameter	3.7 ± 1.0

Alternatively, the spleen index (SI) can be used as a quantitative marker of splenic volume.

SI (cm^2) = transverse diameter (cm) × vertical diameter (cm)

By using a grading system, pathological splenic entities may be deemed more or less likely.

Grade 0 = normal 0–30 cm^2, grade I = mild 31–60 cm^2, grade II = moderate 61–90 cm^2, grade III = marked 91–120 cm^2, and grade IV = marked massive > 120 and massive > 150. No official grade V.

FURTHER READING

Benter T, Kluhs L, Teichgraber U. Sonography of the spleen. *J Ultrasound Med.* 2011; 30:1281–1293.

Frank K, Linhart P, Kortsik C, Wohlenberg H. Sonography in determination of spleen size: Standard dimensions in healthy adults. *Ultraschall in Med.* 1986; 7:134–137.

Hosey RG, Mattacola CG, Kriss V. Ultrasound assessment of spleen size in collegiate athletes. *Br J Sports Med.* 2006; 40:251–254.

Ishibashi H, Higuchi N, Shimamura R, et al. Sonographic assessment and grading of spleen size. *J Clin Ultrasound.* 1991; 19:21–25.

Loftus WK, Metreweli C. Normal splenic size in a Chinese population. *J Ultrasound Med.* 1997; 16:345–347.

Niederau C, Sonnenberg A, Muller JE, Erckenbrecht JF, Scholten T, Fritsch WP. Sonographic measurements of the normal liver, spleen, pancreas, and portal vein. *Radiology.* 1983; 149:537–540.

Rosenberg HK, Markowitz RI, Kolberg H, Park C, Hubbard A, Bell RD. Normal splenic size in infants and children: Sonographic measurements. *AJR Am J Roentgenol.* 1991; 157:119–121.

Pancreas

PREPARATION
Patient should fast for 6–8 hours prior to examination.

POSITION
Supine.

TRANSDUCER
2.0–6.0 MHz curvilinear transducer.

METHOD
If the pancreas is obscured by air, visualization may be improved by drinking 500 ml of water in the right decubitus position. The water bolus outlines the pancreatic head. Longitudinal and transverse images are obtained using the upper abdominal blood vessels as landmarks.

The **pancreatic head** is measured above the inferior vena cava.

The **pancreatic neck** is measured over the superior mesenteric vein.

The **pancreatic body** is measured over the superior mesenteric artery.

APPEARANCE
The pancreas should appear homogenous with a reflectivity greater than or equal to the adjacent liver. Variations in reflectivity relate to the degree of fatty infiltration. After 60 years of age, fat accumulation in pancreatic tissues is common and reflectivity therefore increases. Measurements are relative, and structural abnormalities are more important than absolute dimensions.

MEASUREMENTS

	Transverse anteroposterior diameter (mm)
Pancreatic head	19–25
Pancreatic body	15–20
Pancreatic tail	20–25

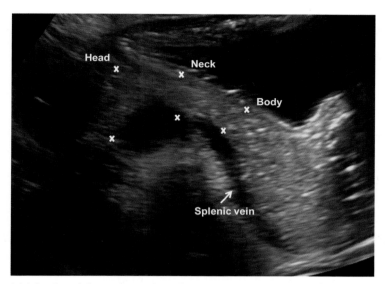

Axial view through the pancreas at the confluence of the splenic vein and superior mesenteric vein. The head, neck, and body are measured on this view.

FURTHER READING

Glaser J, Stienecker K. Pancreas and aging: A study using ultrasonography. *Gerontology*. 2000; 46:93–96.

Pirri C, Cui XW, De Molo C, Ignee A, Schreiber-Dietrich DG, Dietrich CF. The pancreatic head is larger than often assumed. *Z Gastroenterol*. 2013; 51:390–394.

Sienz M, Ignee A, Dietrich CF. Reference values in abdominal ultrasound: Biliopancreatic system and spleen. *Z Gastroenterol*. 2011; 49:845–870.

Sirli R, Sporea I. Ultrasound examination of the normal pancreas. *Med Ultrason*. 2010; 12:62–65.

Pancreatic duct (adult)

PREPARATION
None.

POSITION
Supine.

TRANSDUCER
2.0–5.0 MHz curvilinear transducer.

METHOD
The long axis of the pancreas should be determined. The duct in the region of the head–neck and body is obtained in the transverse/oblique planes. The diameter of the duct is taken as the distance between the inner layers of the anterior and posterior walls.

APPEARANCE
The duct appears as a low reflective tubular structure with reflective walls. The lumen of the pancreatic duct is usually largest in the head of the pancreas and gradually decreases distally.

MEASUREMENTS

| | Normal pancreatic duct diameter (mm) | |
	Range	Mean
Head/neck	2.8–3.3	3
Proximal body	2.0–2.4	2.1
Distal body	1.0–1.7	1.6

The size of the pancreatic duct increases with age, with the upper limit of normal estimated at 3 mm. Administration of secretin causes pancreatic duct dilatation in normal subjects, but has no effect on dilatation caused by chronic pancreatitis and may be used to distinguish these two entities. The diameter of the pancreatic duct can increase during deep inspiration in adults without pancreatic disease, up to 1.3 mm when compared with images obtained at end-expiration.

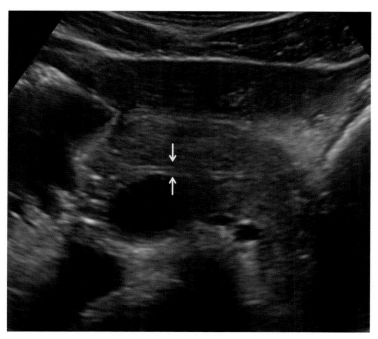

Transverse image of the pancreas to measure the anteroposterior diameter of the pancreatic duct in the proximal aspect of the body.

FURTHER READING

Glaser J, Hogemann B, Krummenerl T, Schneider M, Hultsch E, van Husen N, Gerlach U. Sonographic imaging of the pancreatic duct. New diagnostic possibilities using secretin stimulation. *Digestive Dis Sci.* 1987; 32:1075–1081.

Hadidi A. Pancreatic duct diameter: Sonographic measurement in normal subjects. *J Clin Ultrasound.* 1983; 11:17–22.

Sienz M, Ignee A, Dietrich CF. Reference values in abdominal ultrasound—biliopancreatic system and spleen. *Z Gastroenterol.* 2011; 49:845–870.

Wachsberg RH. Respiratory variation of the diameter of the pancreatic duct on sonography. *AJR Am J Roentgenol.* 2000; 175:1459–1461.

Adrenal glands (adult)

PREPARATION
None.

POSITION
Supine.

TRANSDUCER
2.0–6.0 MHz curvilinear transducer.

METHOD
Anterior transverse images in quiet respiration. The entire gland is not likely to be seen in a single plane of imaging due to the shape of the gland (triangular or crescentic).

The right adrenal gland is best imaged with the patient supine or left lateral decubitus using an intercostal or subcostal approach in the mid-anterior axillary line.

The left adrenal gland is more difficult to see, often due to gas within the stomach. A right lateral decubitus position, using an intercostal approach in the mid- or posterior axillary line, is favored. If a thin patient is imaged supine with deep inspiration, the left adrenal may be seen posterior to the splenic vein.

APPEARANCE
Variable, but an adrenal mass appears as a homogeneous area with a distinct capsule.

The adrenal gland cortex tends to be hypoechoic and the medulla may sometimes be seen as a thin hyperechoic stripe, particularly in younger patients with a resultant "trilaminar" appearance.

The visualization of normal adrenal glands is variable and dependent on operator experience; 78.5%–92% on the right and 44%–71% on the left.

The left gland tends to be more crescentic and the right more triangular, but shapes are variable.

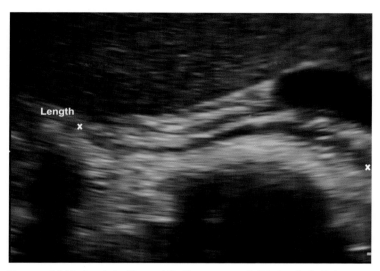

The normal right adrenal gland in an adult with measurement of the length of a limb demonstrated.

MEASUREMENTS

Thickness	0.2–0.8 cm
Length	4–6 cm
Width	2–3 cm

FURTHER READING

Kim KW, Kim JK, Choi HJ. Sonography of the adrenal glands in the adult. *J Clin Ultrasound*. 2012; 40:357–363.

Marchal G, Gelin J, Verbeken E, Baert A, Lauwerijns J. High resolution real-time sonography of the adrenals glands: A routine examination? *J Ultrasound Med*. 1986; 5:65–68

Yeh HC. Sonography of the adrenal glands: Normal glands and small masses. *AJR Am J Roentgenol*. 1980; 135:1167–1177.

Zappasodi F, Derchi LE, Rizzato G. Ultrasonography of the normal adrenal glands: Study using linear array real-time equipment. *Br J Radiol*. 1986; 59:759–764.

Diaphragm

PREPARATION
None.

POSITION
Supine.

TRANSDUCER
2.0–6.0 MHz curvilinear transducer.

METHOD
Performed from a subcostal position, in a longitudinal plane. A cursor is placed at the position of the dome of either the left or right hemidiaphragm at end tidal volume, and then marked at full inspiration. If forced expiration is used, the dome of the diaphragm may not be visible.

APPEARANCE
The thin, high-reflective diaphragmatic curve is readily identified.

MEASUREMENTS
Diaphragm paralysis is demonstrated on B-Mode ultrasound by absent or minimal thickening (< 20%) during inspiration.

	Diaphragm thickness	Diaphragm movement
Normal (quiet) inspiration	2.8 mm	2.2 cm
Deep inspiration	4 mm or more	5.4 cm male 4.0 cm female

M-Mode ultrasound has been shown to be more accurate and reproducible for assessing hemidiaphragmatic movement. Excursions are larger in men. Lower limits are shown below.

	Men	Women
Quiet breathing	1 cm	0.9 cm
Voluntary sniffing	1.8 cm	1.6 cm
Deep breathing	4.7 cm	3.7 cm

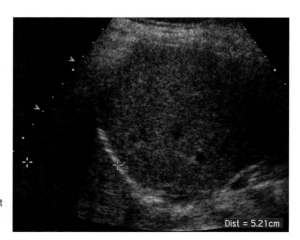

A cursor is placed at the position of the dome of the right hemidiaphragm at end tidal volume, and then marked at full inspiration with a second cursor.

FURTHER READING

Baria MR, Shahgholi L, Sorenson EJ, Harper CJ, Lim KG, Strommen JA, Mottram CD, Boon AJ. B-Mode ultrasound assessment of diaphragm structure and function in patients with COPD. *Chest.* 2014; 146:680–685.

Boussuges A, Gole Y, Blanc P. Diaphragmatic motion studied by M-mode ultrasonography: Methods, reproducibility, and normal values. *Chest.* 2009; 135:391–400.

Harris RS, Giovannetti M, Kim BK. Normal ventilatory movement of the right hemidiaphragm studied by ultrasonography and pneumotachograph. *Radiology.* 1983; 146:141–144.

Houston JG, Morris AD, Howie CA, Reid JL, McMillan N. Technical report: Quantitative assessment of diaphragmatic movement—A reproducible method using ultrasound. *Clin Radiol.*1992; 46:40–47.

Smargiassi A, Inchingolo R, Soldati G, Copetti R, Marchetti G, Zanforlin A, Giannuzzi R, Testa A, Nardini S, Valente S. The role of chest ultrasonography in the management of respiratory diseases: Document II. *Multidiscip Respir Med.* 2013; 8:55.

Testa A, Soldati G, Giannuzzi R, Berardi S, Portale G, Gentiloni Silveri N. Ultrasound M-Mode assessment of diaphragmatic kinetics by anterior transverse scanning in healthy subjects. *Ultrasound Med Biol.* 2011; 37:44–52

Portal vein

PREPARATION
Patient should fast for 4–6 hours prior to the examination.

POSITION
Supine and right anterior oblique.

TRANSDUCER
2.0–6.0 MHz curvilinear transducer.

METHOD
Right longitudinal intercostal approach.

APPEARANCE
Tubular structure in the porta hepatis, branching into the right and left portal veins.

MEASUREMENTS
Normal portal venous velocity varies in the same individual, increasing after a meal and decreasing after exercise. The diameter is measured at the broadest point just distal to the union of the splenic and superior mesenteric vein, normally measuring 11 ± 2 mm. Color and spectral Doppler imaging demonstrates the portal venous system to be an isolated vascular unit with a relatively monophasic flow pattern with fluctuations with cardiac or respiratory movements. Portal venous flow may be pulsatile in healthy subjects and is inversely related to body mass index. In such cases, care should be taken to not attribute pulsatile flow to right heart dysfunction. The Valsalva maneuver results in portal vein dilatation.

Normal portal vein velocity ranges from 16–40 cm/sec.

The congestion index (CI) of the portal vein is determined as follows:

$$\text{Portal vein area} = \text{diameter A} \times \text{diameter B} \times \pi/4$$

$$\text{Flow velocity} = 0.57 \times \text{maximum portal vein velocity (angle} \leq 60°)$$

$$\text{CI} = \text{vein area/flow velocity}$$

The normal value for the CI is 0.070 ± 0.029 cm/sec and increases to 0.171 ± 0.075 cm/sec in patients with portal hypertension.

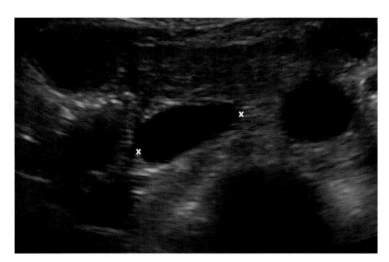

The diameter of the portal vein is measured at the broadest point just distal to the union of the splenic and superior mesenteric vein.

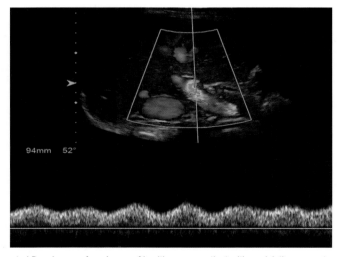

94mm 52°

A spectral Doppler waveform image of healthy young patient with modulation present.

Findings diagnostic for portal hypertension:**
- Low portal venous velocity, < 16 cm/sec
- Hepatofugal portal venous flow
- Dilated portal vein
- Portosystemic shunts, e.g., recanalized umbilical vein

FURTHER READING

Al-Nakshabandi NA. The role of ultrasonography in portal hypertension. *Saudi J Gastroenterol.* 2006; 12:111–117.

Gallix BP, Taourel P, Dauzat M, Brue JMl, Lafortune M. Pulsatility in the portal venous system: A study of Doppler sonography in healthy adults. *AJR Am J Roentgenol.* 1996; 169:141–144.

Görg C, Riera-Knorrenschild J, Dietrich J. Pictorial review: Colour Doppler ultrasound flow patterns in the portal venous system. *Br J Radiol.* 2002; 75:919–929.

McNaughton DA, Abu-Yousef MM. Doppler US of the liver made simple. *Radiographics.* 2011; 31:161–188.

Moriyasu F, Nishida O, Ban N, Nakamura T, Sakai M, Miyake T, Uchino H. "Congestion Index" of the portal vein. *AJR Am J Roentgenol.* 1986; 146:735–739.

Weinreb J, Kumari S, Phillips G, Pochaczevsky R. Portal vein measurements by real-time sonography. *AJR Am J Roentgenol* 1982; 139:497–499.

Hepatic veins

PREPARATION
None.

POSITION
Supine and right anterior oblique.

TRANSDUCER
2.0–6.0 MHz curvilinear transducer.

METHOD
Right lateral intercostal approach during quiet respiration. Place spectral Doppler gate halfway along length of the hepatic vein.

APPEARANCE
There are usually three main hepatic veins (left, middle, and right), but many patients have an accessory or inferior right hepatic vein. These join centrally into the inferior vena cava (IVC) immediately inferior to the diaphragm. Pulsatility within the left hepatic vein is greater than in the middle vein, which is greater than in the right vein, due to transmitted pulsations from the heart. To minimize this effect, the right hepatic vein is normally used for Doppler studies.

MEASUREMENTS
Doppler spectral flow shows a triphasic waveform with two periods of forward flow within each cardiac cycle (corresponding to the two phases of right atrial filling) and the one period of normal, transient reversed flow due to contraction of the right side of the heart. This triphasic pattern alters in cirrhosis, becoming biphasic and eventually monophasic in advanced disease. Pattern alterations are also observed in heart failure and tricuspid regurgitation.

FURTHER READING
Abu-Yousef MM. Duplex Doppler sonography of the hepatic vein in tricuspid regurgitation. *AJR Am J Roentgenol.* 1991; 156:79–83.

Bolondi L, Li Bassi S, Gaiani S, Zironi G, Benzi G, Santi V, Barbara L. Liver cirrhosis: Changes of Doppler waveform of hepatic veins. *Radiology.* 1991; 178:513–516.

Desser TS, Sze DY, Jeffrey RB. Imaging and intervention in the hepatic veins. *AJR Am J Roentgenol.* 2003; 180:1583–1591.

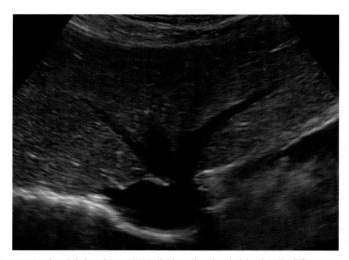

Transverse subcostal view demonstrates the hepatic veins draining into the IVC.

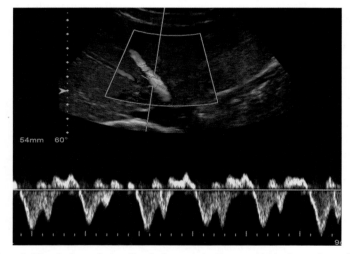

A spectral Doppler trace of a hepatic vein demonstrates the normal triphasic waveform with two periods of forward flow and one period of transient flow within each cardiac cycle.

Farrant P, Meire HB. Hepatic vein pulsatility assessment on spectral Doppler ultrasound (short communication). *Br J Radiol.* 1997; 70:829–832.

Hepatic artery

PREPARATION
None.

POSITION
Supine and right anterior oblique.

TRANSDUCER
2.0–6.0 MHz curvilinear transducer.

METHOD
Right oblique intercostal approach. Locate the celiac axis anterior to the aorta and then follow the arterial branch that runs to the right.

APPEARANCE
The hepatic artery originates as one of the three major branches of the celiac axis, lying anteromedial to the portal vein at the porta hepatis. In 50% there is some anatomic variation or aberrant origin of the artery, either an accessory or more commonly a replaced artery. On the right, the superior mesenteric artery most commonly gives rise to the aberrant artery, often dorsal to the portal vein.

The hepatic arterial waveform is typically pulsatile with low resistance.

The hepatic artery is located adjacent to the portal vein, and a spectral Doppler trace demonstrates the resistance waveform pattern.

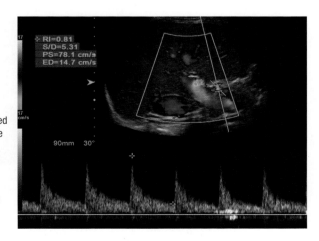

MEASUREMENTS

Resistance index (RI): Measured as the proper hepatic artery crosses the portal vein.

$$RI = \frac{\text{Peak Systolic Velocity} - \text{End Diastolic Velocity}}{\text{Peak Systolic Velocity}}$$

RI of the normal hepatic artery ranges from 0.55–0.81.

Causes of high RI	Causes of low RI
Post-prandial state	Proximal stenosis, e.g., at transplant vessel anastomosis
Advanced patient age	Distal vascular shunting
Chronic liver disease, e.g., cirrhosis, chronic hepatitis	Cirrhosis with portal hypertension
Downstream stenosis	Upstream stenosis (causing tardus parvus waveform)
Transplant rejection	Trauma

Patients with colorectal hepatic metastases have significantly greater arterial blood flow and Doppler perfusion index (DPI) and reduced portovenous flow.

DPI of the hepatic artery is calculated as follows:

$$DPI = \frac{\text{Hepatic arterial flow}}{\text{Total liver blood flow}}$$

(Total liver blood flow = Hepatic arterial blood flow and portal venous blood flow; Blood flow = time-average velocity of blood vessel × time-average cross-sectional area of lumen of vessel.)

The upper limit of the normal range of DPI values is 0.25. Benign lesions may have a DPI ranging from 0.05–0.53, while malignant lesions demonstrate a DPI from 0.39–0.75.

FURTHER READING

Grant EG, Schiller VL, Millener P, Tessler FN, Perrella RR, Ragavendra N, Busuttil R. Color Doppler imaging of the hepatic vasculature. *AJR Am J Roentgenol*. 1992; 159:943–950.

Joynt LK, Platt JF, Rubin JM, Ellis JH, Bude RO. Hepatic artery resistance before and after standard meal. Subjects with diseased and healthy livers. *Radiology*. 1995; 196:489–492.

Kopljar M, Brkljacic B, Doko M, Horzic M. Nature of Doppler perfusion index changes in patients with colorectal cancer liver metastases. *J Ultrasound Med*. 2004; 23:1295–1300.

Kyriakopoulou K, Antoniou A, Fezoulidis IV, Kelekis NL, Dalekos GN, Vlychou M. The role of Doppler Perfusion Index as screening test in the characterization of focal liver lesions. *Dig Liver Dis*. 2008; 40:755–760.

Leen E, Goldberg JA, Robertson J, Angerson WJ, Sutherland GR, Cooke TG, McArdle CS. Early detection of occult colorectal metastases using duplex colour Doppler sonography. *Br J Surg*. 1993; 80:1249–1251.

McNaughton DA, Abu-Yousef MM. Doppler US of the liver made simple. *Radiographics*. 2011; 31:161–188.

Celiac and superior mesenteric arteries

PREPARATION
Patient should fast for 8–12 hours prior to the examination.

POSITION
Patient supine.

TRANSDUCER
1.0–5.0 MHz curvilinear transducer.

METHOD
Ensure a Doppler beam/vessel angle of ≤ 60°. Locate the level of the supra-renal aorta in the transverse plane, identifying the celiac artery (CA) and the superior mesenteric artery (SMA), and then examine in the longitudinal direction. Use a sample volume of 2 mm. Measure the peak systolic velocity (PSV) as the sample volume is moved from the aorta to the proximal arteries. Record the maximum peak systolic velocity.

APPEARANCE
Best seen in the longitudinal view, where the CA and SMAs arise from the anterior aspect of the aorta, in close proximity to each other. Only high-grade mesenteric artery stenosis (≥ 70%) are likely to be symptomatic.

MEASUREMENTS
PSVs show a higher overall accuracy than end diastolic velocity (EDV).

	Superior mesenteric artery PSV (cm/s)	Celiac axis PSV (cm/s)
Normal	125 ± 25	123 ± 27
Stenosis ≥ 50%	295	240
Stenosis ≥ 70%	400	320

FURTHER READING
AbuRahma AF, Stone PA, Srivastava M, Dean LS Keiffer T Hass SM, Mousa AY. Mesenteric/celiac duplex ultrasound interpretation criteria revisited. *J Vascular Surg.* 2012; 55:428–436.

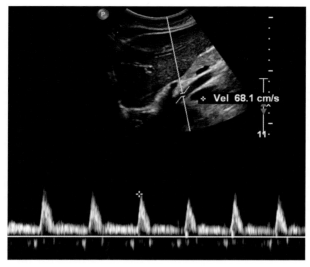

Peak systolic velocity in the proximal SMA. Angle correction is imprecise in the proximal SMA if there is significant curvature.

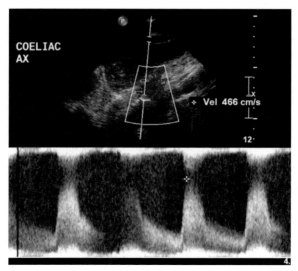

High velocities in the CA origin indicate a severe stenosis.

Doppler ultrasound measurement of post-prandial intestinal blood flow

PREPARATION
Patient should fast overnight, and the examination should be performed after 30 minutes of supine rest.

POSITION
Patient supine with head of bed elevated 30°.

TRANSDUCER
1.0–5.0 MHz curvilinear transducer.

METHOD
Superior mesenteric and celiac arteries can be identified either longitudinally or transversely. The angle of insonation should be kept at ≤ 60° and the vessels examined along their visible length. The following parameters may be measured: peak systolic velocity (PSV), end diastolic velocity (EDV), and the pulsatility index (PI). A "standard" 800 kcal meal is consumed and serial Doppler measurements are made over the following hour.

$$PI = \frac{\text{Peak Systolic Velocity} - \text{End Diastolic Velocity}}{\text{Time averaged maximum velocity}}$$

APPEARANCE
Best seen in the longitudinal view, where the celiac axis and superior mesenteric arteries arise from the anterior aspect of the aorta, in close proximity to each other.

MEASUREMENTS

	Pre-meal			Post-meal		
	Superior mesenteric artery					
	PSV	**EDV**	**PI**	**PSV**	**EDV**	**PI**
Normal	100 cm/s	16 cm/s	3.6	154 cm/s	46 cm/s	1.8
	Celiac axis					
Normal	120 cm/s	30 cm/s	1.5	130 cm/s	40 cm/s	1.5

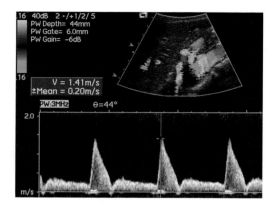

The superior mesenteric artery spectral Doppler waveform in a fasting patient.

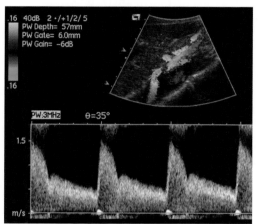

The spectral Doppler waveform has altered following a meal, with a high forward diastolic component.

A meal should cause an increase in both systolic and diastolic velocities and a reduction in the PI, indicative of a fall in distal mesenteric vascular impedance. The increase in superior mesenteric artery EDV can be between 150% and 300%. Changes in the celiac artery are less noticeable as the bulk of celiac blood flow is not to the gut.

FURTHER READING

Muller AF, Role of duplex Doppler ultrasound in the assessment of patients with postprandial abdominal pain. *Gut.* 1992; 33:460–465.

Inferior mesenteric artery

PREPARATION
Patient should fast overnight.

POSITION
Supine.

TRANSDUCER
1.0–5.0 MHz curvilinear transducer or 3–8 MHz linear array transducer.

METHOD
The inferior mesenteric artery (IMA) is identified arising from the aorta anteriorly and to the left. Spectral Doppler waveforms are obtained from the proximal 3–4 cm of the artery along its longitudinal axis (Doppler angle ≤ 60°). The IMA is seen in 92% of subjects.

APPEARANCE
Tubular structure arising from the aorta.

MEASUREMENTS
The spectral Doppler waveform demonstrates pulsatile flow that may be triphasic. Stenosis of the IMA is diagnosed by velocity increase.

Normal values
PSV 98 ± 30 cm/s
EDV 11 ± 5 cm/s

Optimum threshold for stenosis ≥ 50%
PSV ≥ 250 cm/s
EDV ≥ 90 cm/s
IMA/Aortic PSV ratio ≥4

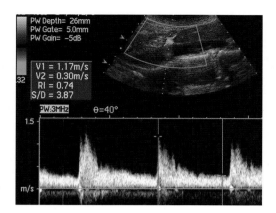

A longitudinal image through the lower aorta demonstrates the inferior mesenteric artery.

FURTHER READING

AbuRahma AF, Dean LS. Duplex ultrasound interpretation criteria for inferior mesenteric arteries. *Vascular.* 2012; 20: 145–149.

Denys AL, Lafortune M, Aubin B, Burke M, Breton G. Doppler sonography of the inferior mesenteric artery: A preliminary study. *J Ultrasound Med.* 1995; 14:435–439.

Erden A, Yurdakul M, Cumhur T. Doppler waveforms of the normal and collateralized inferior mesenteric artery. *AJR Am J Roentgeneol.* 1998; 171:619–627.

2 URINARY TRACT

Venus Hedayati, Colin R. Deane,
Keshthra Satchithananda, and
Paul S. Sidhu

Kidneys

PREPARATION
None.

POSITION
Supine, left and right anterior oblique and, if necessary, prone.

TRANSDUCER
2.0–6.0 MHz curvilinear transducer.
Tissue harmonic imaging is often used, particularly in obese patients.

METHOD
Image the right kidney using the liver as an acoustic window. The left kidney is typically more difficult to visualize. The left anterior oblique 45° or right decubitus position may help, and asking the patient to suspend respiration ensures less movement. Both kidneys should be imaged in both longitudinal and transverse planes.
To better visualize the upper poles, ipsilateral arm elevation and deep inspiration may be useful.
The right kidney lies 1–2 cm lower than the left.

APPEARANCE
The kidneys comprise three main parts: the cortex, the sinus, and the medulla.

The cortex comprises the bulk of the kidney, and reflectivity of the renal cortex is less than the adjacent spleen on the left and either slightly less reflective or isoechoic to the liver on the right. The renal sinus contains multiple structures—the pelvis, calyces, vessels, and fat—and is hyper-echoic due to the presence of fat. The renal pyramids (medulla) are poorly defined triangular structures at the outer edge of the renal sinus at regular junctions with the cortex and are hypo-echoic. The renal capsule can be identified as a thin, high-reflective rim.

MEASUREMENTS
Three measurements can be made and a volume calculated (0.49 × Length × Width × Anterior Posterior diameter), although usually, only a length is required.

Length: Obtained from the sagittal image, measuring the longest cranio-caudal length. This is usually the only quoted measurement in a report.

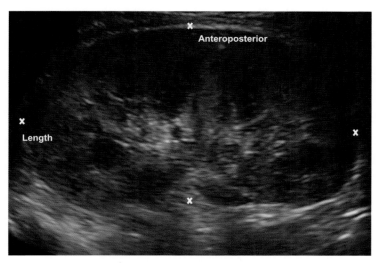

A sagittal image with two measurements obtained in the longitudinal and anteroposterior directions.

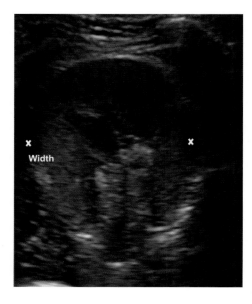

The width is measured from a transverse image obtained through the renal hilum.

Anteroposterior dimension: Measured from the sagittal image measured perpendicular to the long axis.

Width: Measured from a transverse image taken from the lateral margin of the kidney through the renal hilum.

Renal cortical thickness is >1 cm over the pyramids, but that measurement often decreases with age.

Renal length decreases with age, almost entirely as a result of parenchymal reduction. Height and age, but not sex, are determinate of renal size. There is no difference in kidney length measurements in the supine oblique and prone positions.

Normal mean values in cm (± SD)*

		Length	Anteroposterior	Width
Right kidney	Oblique	10.65 ± 1.4	3.95 ± 0.8	4.92 ± 0.6
	Prone	10.74 ± 1.4	4.17 ± 0.5	5.05 ± 0.8
Left kidney	Oblique	10.13 ± 1.2	3.58 ± 0.9	5.30 ± 0.7
	Prone	11.10 ± 1.2	4.14 ± 0.8	5.30 ± 0.8

Size of the kidney with age in cm (decades)^

	3rd	4th	5th	6th	7th	8th	9th
Right	11.3	11.2	11.2	11.0	10.7	9.9	9.6
Left	11.5	11.5	11.4	11.3	10.9	10.2	9.8

FURTHER READING

*Brandt TD, Nieman HL, Dragowski MJ, Bulawa W, Claykamp G. Ultrasound assessment of normal renal dimension. *J Ultrasound Med.* 1982; 1:49–52.

Emamian SA, Nielsen MB, Pedersen JF, Ytte L. Kidney dimensions at sonography: Correlation with age, sex, and habitus in 665 adult volunteers. *AJR Am J Roentgenol.* 1993;160:83-86.

^Miletic D, Fuckar Z, Sustic A, Mozetic V, Stimac D, Zauhar G. Sonographic measurement of absolute and relative renal length in adults. *J Clin Ultrasound.* 1998; 26:185–189.

Evaluation of acute renal obstruction with intrarenal Doppler

PREPARATION
None.

POSITION
Supine.

TRANSDUCER
2.0–6.0 MHz curvilinear transducer.

METHOD
Doppler signals are obtained from arcuate arteries at the corticomedullary junction or interlobar arteries along the border of medullary pyramids. The Doppler waveforms should be made on the lowest pulse repetition frequency without aliasing to maximize the size of the Doppler spectrum. The Resistance Index (RI) is calculated from the formula:

$$RI = \frac{\text{Peak Systolic Velocity} - \text{End Diastolic Velocity}}{\text{Peak Systolic Velocity}}$$

APPEARANCE
The normal spectral Doppler waveforms in the renal arcuate arteries are those of a low-resistance end-organ, with a broad systolic peak and an elevated end-diastolic velocity.

MEASUREMENTS
Elevation of the RI occurs after just 6 hours of clinical obstruction.

Mean RI in normal kidneys is 0.60 ± 0.04.

Mean RI of obstructed kidneys is 0.77 ± 0.07.

If there is pyelosinus extravasation on the urographic imaging or the duration of obstruction is less than 6 hours, the RI may not be elevated.

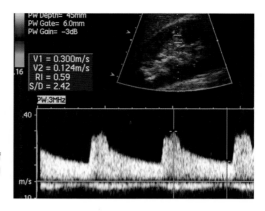

PW Depth= 45mm
PW Gate= 6.0mm
PW Gain= -3dB

V1 = 0.300m/s
V2 = 0.124m/s
RI = 0.59
S/D = 2.42
PW:3MHz

Doppler signals are obtained from the arcuate arteries at the corticomedullary junction of the interlobar arteries along the border of the medullary pyramids.

FURTHER READING

Platt JF, Rubin JM, Ellis JH. Acute renal obstruction: Evaluation with intrarenal duplex Doppler and conventional US. *Radiology.* 1993; 186:685–688.

Rodgers PM, Bates JA, Irving HC. Intrarenal Doppler studies in normal and acutely obstructed kidneys. *Br J Radiol.* 1992; 65:207–212.

Renal circulation and renal artery

PREPARATION
None.

POSITION
Supine, lateral decubitus.

TRANSDUCER
Low-frequency curvilinear (typically 1.0–5.0 MHz). A low-frequency phased array (1.0–4.0 MHz) may be useful to investigate the renal artery.

METHOD

Intrarenal arteries
The kidneys are imaged from the flank with the patient in a supine or lateral decubitus position. Coronal views usually give a clear longitudinal image of the kidneys, although there is anatomical variation and oblique views may be better. The liver and spleen can be used as acoustic windows. For intrarenal arteries, a higher color frequency (typically 3 MHz) gives greater sensitivity to segmental and interlobar arteries. For intrarenal arteries, angle correction is usually not required because the resistance index (RI) is the main measurement taken.

Renal arteries
The proximal renal arteries can be obtained from an anterior transverse view. This usually offers a clear B-mode image of the renal artery origins. Color Doppler frequency should be low (2 MHz). The Doppler angle correction should be ≤ 60°.

The renal arteries may also be imaged from the patient's flank in a coronal or oblique view, although transverse views may be useful. This view often allows images of the entire renal artery to segmental artery level. Doppler angle corrections are usually low because the renal arteries are closely aligned to the beam direction. Velocities measured in this view may be lower than angle-corrected measurements from an anterior approach.

Velocities should be measured from origin to segmental artery level and the highest velocity obtained. Atherosclerotic renal artery stenosis is usually at the ostium and proximal renal artery; fibromuscular dysplasia stenosis is usually in the mid/distal renal artery.

APPEARANCE

Appearances as described above.

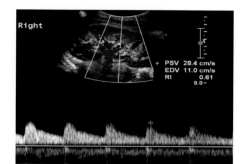

Intrarenal flow waveform from a healthy kidney showing low resistance flow with a RI of 0.61.

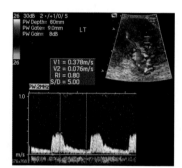

Increased renovascular resistance results in a loss of diastolic flow measured as an RI of 0.8.

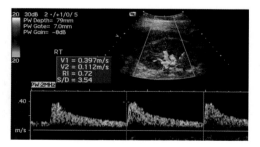

Slow heart rates result in a longer diastolic phase with a reduction in end diastolic flow. This increases RI. With a faster heart rate, the RI would be less than 0.72 measured here.

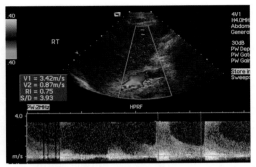

High velocities in the renal artery origin indicates a tight stenosis. There is no beam/flow angle correction made, so peak systolic velocity (PSV) is at least 342 cm/s. Problems when measuring renal artery velocities include movement through the sample volume and the need for high pulse repetition frequency with an additional sample volume and reduced signal/noise in the sonogram.

MEASUREMENTS

Intrarenal arteries

$$\text{Resistance Index (RI)} = \frac{\text{Peak Systolic Velocity} - \text{End Diastolic Velocity}}{\text{Peak Systolic Velocity}}$$

The RI in healthy kidneys ranges from 0.55–0.7, increasing with age. There is variation within a kidney; flow waveforms in healthy kidneys become less pulsatile from the renal artery through to the interlobar and distal artery level. RI should be measured at the interlobar artery level for consistency.

Resistance indices of ≥ 0.8 are associated with reduced renal blood flow and increased renovascular resistance in a range of parenchymal disorders. Resistance indices of 1.0 are associated with severely impaired renal function.

Care should be taken when reporting RIs in patients with low heart rates. The long diastolic component results in reduced end diastolic flows and elevated RIs.

Renal arteries

The normal PSV in adult renal arteries is from 60–100 cm/s; it is slightly higher in children. Peak velocities of ≥ 180 cm/s are indicative of stenosis; velocities ≥ 200 cm/s have been shown to have good correlation with pressure drops of 20 mmHg with higher velocities indicative of more severe disease. Renal artery–aortic ratio (RAR) of > 3.0 is indicative of stenosis, with higher values more specific of stenosis.

Intrarenal flow waveform changes have been proposed as indicative of stenosis. Most commonly used is an acceleration time of > 70 ms. Several studies have shown this to have high specificity but low sensitivity to stenosis.

FURTHER READING

House MK, Dowling RJ, King P, Gibson RN. Using Doppler sonography to reveal renal artery stenosis: An evaluation of optimal imaging parameters. *AJR Am J Roentgenol.* 1999; 173:761–765.

Kawarda O, Yokoi Y, Takemoto K, Morioka N, Nakata S, Shiotani S. The performance of renal duplex ultrasonography for the detection of hemodynamically significant renal artery stenosis. *Cath Cardiovasc Intervent.* 2006; 68: 311–318.

Keogan MT, Kliewer MA, Hertzberg BS, DeLong DM, Tupler RH, Carroll BA. Renal resistive indexes: Variability in Doppler US measurement in a healthy population. *Radiology.* 1996; 199:165–169.

Staub D, Canevascini R, Huegli RW, Aschwanden M, Thalhammer C, Imfeld S, Singer E, Jacob AL, Jaeger KA. Best duplex-sonographic criteria for the assessment of renal artery stenosis—correlation with intra-arterial pressure gradient. *Ultraschall Med.* 2007; 28:45–51.

Tublin ME, Bude RO, Platt JF. The resistive index in renal Doppler sonography: Where do we stand? *AJR Am J Roentgenol.* 2003; 180:885–892.

Retroperitoneal lymph nodes

PREPARATION
None.

POSITION
Supine.

TRANSDUCER
2.0–6.0 MHz curvilinear transducer

METHOD
Longitudinal and transverse sections are used to image the aorta and the inferior vena cava. Lymph nodes can sometimes be identified around these structures. In normal subjects and with adequate visualization, normal-sized lymph nodes are most likely to be detected, in descending order of frequency, in the aorto-caval, left para-aortic, and peripancreatic regions.

APPEARANCE
Normal lymph nodes are flattened, low-reflective structures with an eccentric highly reflective area representing the fatty hilum.

MEASUREMENT
Lymph nodes > 1 cm short axis are considered to be abnormally enlarged.

FURTHER READING

Dietrich CF, Zeuzem S, Caspary WF, Wehrmann T. Ultrasound lymph node imaging in the abdomen and retroperitoneum of health probands. *Ultraschall in Medizin*. 1998; 19:265–269.

Koenigsberg M, Hoffman JC, Schnur J. Sonographic evaluation of the retroperitoneum. *Sem Ultrasound*. 1982; 3:79–96.

Marchal G, Oyen R, Verschakelen J, Gelin J, Baert AL, Stessens RC. Sonographic appearance of normal lymph nodes. *J Ultrasound Med*. 1985; 4:417–419.

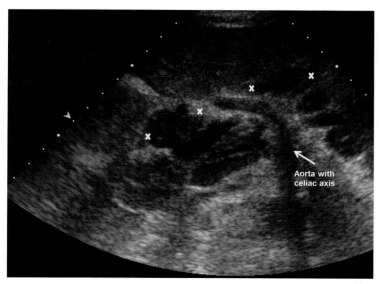

An axial section at the level of the aorta and celiac axia, demonstrating multiple enlarged lymph nodes.

Bladder volume and residual volume

PREPARATION
Patient must have a full bladder.

POSITION
Supine.

TRANSDUCER
3.0–6.0 MHz curvilinear transducer.

METHOD
Transverse plane for the width depth and then a longitudinal image provides the length measurement. Measurements are estimated both pre- and post-micturition.

APPEARANCE
When full, the bladder is clearly defined as an almost square structure of low reflectivity in the transverse plane. Within the bladder the trigone is the area containing the ureteric and urethral orifices. The urethral orifice marks the bladder neck.

MEASUREMENTS
The normal bladder volume when full is approximately 400–500 ml.

$$\text{Bladder Volume (ml)} = \frac{\pi \times \text{Length} \times \text{Depth} \times \text{Width}}{6}$$

($\pi/6$ may be substituted by 0.52)

The accuracy of this calculation is variable, as it is based on an ellipsoid formula, and there is considerable bladder shape variation. At least 200 ml of fluid must be in the bladder to make an urodynamic flow rate study accurate. The normal residual post-micturition volume is < 12 ml in 100% and < 5 ml in 78% of patients. A volume of > 50 ml is usually clinically significant. If there remains a > 100 ml residual volume, the patient should attempt further bladder emptying and the examination should be repeated.

FURTHER READING
Griffiths CJ, Murray A, Ramsden PD. Accuracy and repeatability of bladder volume measurement using ultrasonic imaging. *J Urol.* 1986; 136:808–812.

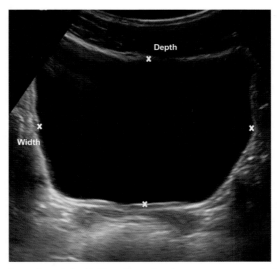

A transverse image through the bladder with an almost square appearance of a full bladder with measurement cursors in position measuring depth and width.

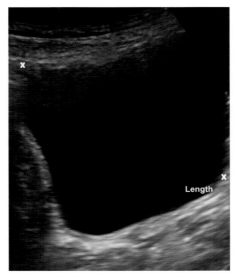

A longitudinal image through the bladder with measurement cursors in position measuring length.

Manieri C, Carter SS, Romano G, Trucchi A, Valenti M, Tubaro A. The diagnosis of bladder outlet obstruction in men by ultrasound measurement of bladder wall thickness. *J Urol*. 1998; 159;761–765.

McLean GK, Edell SL. Determination of bladder volumes by gray scale ultrasonography. *Radiology*. 1978; 128:181–182.

Poston GJ, Joseph AE, Riddle PR. The accuracy of ultrasound in the measurement of changes in bladder volume. *Br J Urol*. 1983; 55:361–363.

Bladder wall

PREPARATION
Patient must have a full bladder.

POSITION
Supine.

TRANSDUCER
3.0–6.0 MHz curvilinear transducer.

METHOD
Bladder wall is measured on transverse and longitudinal images by placing the transducer in the midline above the pubis. The optimal sites for measurement are the bladder floor lateral to the trigone on transverse views and the posterior inferior wall on sagittal views.

APPEARANCE
Smooth contour with the high-reflective mucosa distinguishable from the low reflective detrusor muscle.

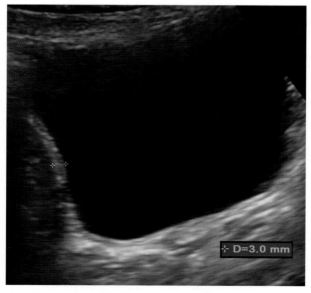

The bladder wall is measured posteriorly at an optimal position.

MEASUREMENTS

Detrusor wall thickness decreases continuously while the bladder fills to 50% of its capacity, usually 250 ml, but then stays constant until filled to 100% capacity. Therefore, measurements should be made when the bladder is full.

Men tend to have a fractionally greater bladder wall thickness. Regardless of the patient's age and body mass index:

Normal empty bladder ≤ 5 mm

Well distended bladder < 2 mm

Global thickening > 5 mm can be a sign of bladder outlet obstruction.

FURTHER READING

Jequier S, Rousseau O. Sonographic measurements of the normal bladder wall in children. *AJR Am J Roentgenol.* 1987; 149:563–566.

Manieri C, Carter SSC, Romano G, Trucchi A, Valenti M, Tubaro A. The diagnosis of bladder outlet obstruction in men by ultrasound measurement of bladder wall thickness. *J Urol.* 1998; 159:761–765.

Oelke M, Höfner K, Wiese B, Grünewald V, Jonas U. Increase in detrusor wall thickness indicates bladder outlet obstruction in men. *World J Urol.* 2002; 19:443–452.

Functional bladder imaging

PREPARATION
The bladder should ideally be comfortably full but distended to < 600 ml to prevent overstretching.

POSITION
Supine for ultrasound imaging. Standing or sitting for flow-rate analysis.

TRANSDUCER
3.0–6.0 MHz curvilinear transducer. A flow meter is required.

METHOD
Combination of bladder ultrasound with flow-rate measurement to analyze bladder function.

After measuring the full bladder capacity and wall thickness, the flow rate can be measured using a flow meter, which records the volume of urine expelled per unit time (ml/s). The patient should be made comfortable for accurate physiological measurements.

A post-micturition volume should then be measured to document residual volumes; a second postvoid residual may be necessary.

APPEARANCE
No imaging needed, except to confirm adequate prevoiding volume and residual postvoiding volume.

MEASUREMENTS
The total voided volume should be at least 150 ml for accurate flowmetry.

Normal flow pattern

Bladder capacity	400–500 ml male 350–500 ml female
Maximal flow rate	15 ml/s >15 ml/s male > 60 years >25 ml/s male < 40 years 30–50 ml/s female
Average flow rate	10 ml/s
Time to maximal flow	10 s or < 1/3 total flow time
Flow time	30 s
Voiding pressure	40–50 cm H_2O male 30–40 cm H_2O female
Post-void residual	< 25 ml

FURTHER READING
Sahdev A. Functional imaging of the bladder. *Imaging*. 2008;
20:147–154.

3

ORGAN TRANSPLANTATION

Anu E. Obaro, Venus Hedayati, Colin R. Deane, Keshthra Satchithananda, and Paul S. Sidhu

Liver transplantation

PREPARATION
None.

POSITION
Supine or right anterior oblique position.

TRANSDUCER
3.0–6.0 MHz curvilinear transducer.

METHOD
Ultrasound is the primary modality for detection and follow-up of vascular complications of hepatic transplantation. Assessment of the liver parenchyma, biliary tree, and vasculature is performed. Longitudinal and transverse images are taken from a subcostal or intercostal approach on inspiration in the supine and right anterior oblique positions.

APPEARANCE
Liver parenchyma should be homogenous or slightly heterogeneous on gray-scale imaging. In the early postoperative period a trace of perihepatic fluid may be present, which commonly resolves within 10 days. The biliary tree should be of normal caliber.

Hepatic artery: Visualized at the porta-hepatis. Normal hepatic artery Doppler waveform shows a rapid systolic upstroke and low-velocity continuous diastolic flow. Complications include hepatic artery thrombosis, which accounts for 60% of posttransplant vascular complications and manifests as absence of hepatic artery and intrahepatic arterial flow. Sometimes flow is detected in the intrahepatic location due to collateral vessel formation. A tardus parvus waveform is a characteristic change in arterial flow distal to a stenosis. Absence of arterial flow at the porta-hepatis with tardus parvus waveform distally within an intrahepatic artery is suggestive of main artery thrombosis. Hepatic artery stenosis most frequently occurs at the anastomotic site and is seen in up to 11% of transplants.

Portal vein: Visualized at porta-hepatis. Normal portal vein Doppler waveform shows continuous flow pattern with mild velocity variations induced by respiration. Complications include portal vein thrombosis and stenosis. Thrombosis may be seen as expansion of the portal vein with intraluminal echogenicity and absence of color Doppler flow, with chronic thrombosis causing portal vein narrowing. Color and spectral Doppler ultrasound shows no detectable flow in the portal vein.

Hepatic veins and inferior vena cava (IVC): Doppler spectral waveforms of the hepatic veins and IVC are similar with phasic flow pattern indicative of physiologic changes in blood flow with cardiac cycle.

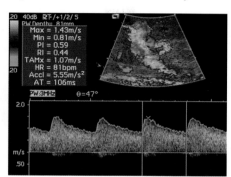

The posttransplant hepatic artery demonstrating a low Resistance Index (RI) estimated at 0.44, and a prolonged acceleration time (AT) indicating the tardus parvus spectral Doppler waveform of a hepatic artery stenosis.

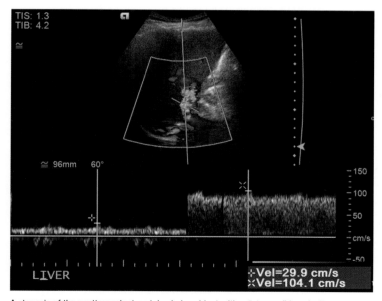

A stenosis of the posttransplant portal vein is evident with a "step-up" in velocity measurements across a focal narrowing, from 29.9 cm/s to 104.1 cm/s.

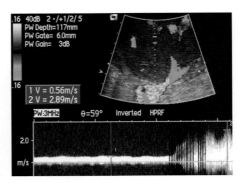

A spectral Doppler gate is placed over the distal hepatic vein at the anastomosis with the suprahepatic inferior vena cava, and an increase in velocity from 0.56 m/s to 2.89 m/s indicates a focal stenosis in the hepatic vein.

MEASUREMENTS

In the posttransplant patient, the normal hepatic arterial Resistance Index (RI) ranges from 0.55–0.80.

$$RI = \frac{\text{Peak Systolic Velocity} - \text{End Diastolic Velocity}}{\text{Peak Systolic Velocity}}$$

Transient high-resistance Doppler waveforms are commonly seen in normal hepatic arteries posttransplant due to decreased diastolic flow. The RI usually normalizes within 7–5 days.

A tardus parvus waveform is a characteristic change in arterial flow distal to a stenosis. This waveform has a RI < 0.5 and a prolonged systolic acceleration time (time from end diastole to first systolic peak) > 0.08 seconds. Hepatic artery stenosis may show narrowing at the anastomotic site on the gray-scale imaging and a focal increase in velocity > 2–3 m/sec with associated turbulence distal to the anastomosis.

Stenosis of the portal vein shows focal color aliasing with a > 3- to 4-fold increase in velocity relative to the pre-stenotic segment, or an absolute velocity measurement of > 100 cm/sec at the site of the stenosis.

Thrombosis or stenosis of IVC can occur after transplantation, and the latter is usually at the site of the anastomosis. Gray-scale ultrasound shows high-reflective thrombus or obvious narrowing. Spectral Doppler evaluation shows a 3- to 4-fold increase in velocity across the stenosis with loss of normal caval phasicity in the hepatic venous spectral Doppler waveform. Loss of phasicity in the hepatic veins also indicates upper caval anastomotic stenosis.

FURTHER READING

Crossin JD, Muradali D, Wilson SR. US of liver transplants: Normal and abnormal. *Radiographics.* 2003; 23:1093–1114.

García-Criado A, Gilabert R, Berzigotti A, Brú C. Doppler ultrasound findings in the hepatic artery shortly after liver transplantation. *AJR Am J Roentgenol.* 2009; 193:128–135.

Renal transplantation

PREPARATION
None.

POSITION
Supine or right anterior oblique position.

TRANSDUCER
1.0–5.0 MHz curvilinear transducer. Alternatively a 3.0–8.0 MHz linear array transducer can be used.

METHOD
Renal transplants are situated in a retroperitoneal position in the iliac fossa. The size may be measured in three planes, to calculate volume. Spectral Doppler waveforms from the upper, mid, and lower aspects are obtained, aided by color Doppler imaging.

APPEARANCE
The transplant kidney may lie in various planes; there may be a prominent pelvi-calyceal system. Corticomedullary differentiation may be readily visualized, and the renal sinus fat is of markedly high reflectivity. The renal pyramids tend to be more readily visualized in a transplant kidney due to decreased echogenicity relative to the rest of the kidney.

Evaluation of the graft alone with B-mode is nonspecific and operator dependent. The gray-scale images should be evaluated with the vascular Doppler findings. In cases without a clear vascular insult, biopsy may be necessary to exclude the underlying cause of graft failure. Perinephric collections can be easily diagnosed and may be a result of hematoma, abscess, urinoma, or lymphoceles.

Graft failure: This may result in nonspecific renal enlargement, cortical thickness increase, changes in renal echogenicity, prominent pyramids, effacement of the renal sinus fat, and loss of corticomedullary differentiation. Focal areas of increased or diminished echogenicity in the graft are also nonspecific and may relate to infarction, infection, or rejection.

Hydronephrosis: Dilated calyces can be due to potential denervation and lack of ureteral tone. If the bladder is full and the calyces are dilated, the patient should fully void and a repeat study should be performed.

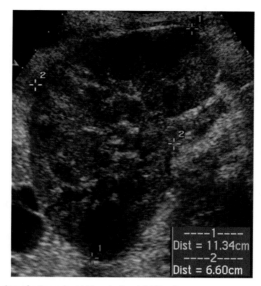

Longitudinal view of a transplant kidney in the right iliac fossa.

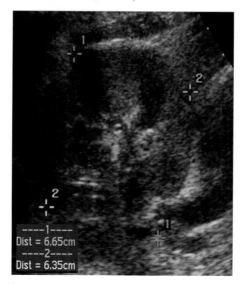

Transverse view of the same transplant kidney, with three measurements obtained to calculate the volume.

Obstruction occurs in 2% of grafts, almost always within 6 months of transplantation, and may be a result of anastomotic edema, ischemic strictures, kinking of the ureter, infection, or obstructive collections.

Exclusion of highly echogenic masses in the collecting system is important to consider in suspected fungal balls, although hematoma and, in the late postoperative stage, tumors can also cause these appearances.

MEASUREMENTS

Volume = 0.49 × Length × Width × Anteroposterior diameter

If < 90% of the immediate postoperative volume, consider chronic rejection or a vascular insult.

Flow waveforms: The Resistance Index (RI) may be measured at the upper, mid, and lower aspects of the transplant kidney, normally from an interlobular branch.

$$RI = \frac{\text{Peak Systolic Velocity} - \text{End Diastolic Velocity}}{\text{Peak Systolic Velocity}}$$

The normal mean value is 0.64–0.73, abnormal if > 0.75, but serial measurement changes over time are more important than single measurements.

FURTHER READING

Absy M, Metreweli C, Matthews C, Al Khader A. Changes in transplanted kidney volume measured by ultrasound. *Br J Radiol.* 1987; 60:525–529.

Don S, Kopecky KK, Filo RS, Leapman SB, Thomalla JV, Jones JA, Klatte EC. Duplex Doppler US of renal allografts. Causes of elevated resistive index. *Radiology.* 1989; 171:709–712.

Hricak H, Lieto RP. Sonographic determination of renal volume. *Radiology.* 1983; 148:311–312.

Rifkin MD, Needleman L, Pasto ME, Kurtz AB, Foy PM, McGlynn E, Canino C, Baltarowich OH, Pennell RG, Goldberg BB. Evaluation of renal transplant rejection by duplex Doppler examination: Value of resistive index. *AJR Am J Roentgenol.* 1987; 148:759–762.

Renal artery stenosis in transplantation

PREPARATION
None.

POSITION
Supine or right anterior oblique position.

PROBE
1.0–5.0 MHz curvilinear transducer.

METHOD
Renal transplants are situated in a retroperitoneal position in the iliac fossa. Doppler spectral analysis is performed along the length of the transplant artery, angle of insonation < 60°, using the lowest filter setting and a scale that accommodates the highest peak systolic velocities without aliasing.

APPEARANCE
The renal artery is sutured end-to-side of the recipient external iliac artery and the renal vein to the external iliac vein. There may be multiple renal arteries. The renal artery may be tortuous, especially in slim recipients where the donor vessels have redundant length.

MEASUREMENTS
Stenosis appears as a focal increase in PSV. A PSV of ≤ 200 cm/sec is usually considered normal. Tortuosity can lead to locally elevated velocities. Thresholds for significant stenosis vary slightly between studies, but ≥ 250 cm/s is recommended as the threshold.

Damped flow waveforms distal to a stenosis, as described by a reduction in Resistance Index (RI) and increased acceleration time (time from the beginning of the systolic upstroke to the first systolic peak) recorded in the intrarenal vessels, are helpful in identifying a proximal stenosis but have poor sensitivity.

$$RI = \frac{\text{Peak Systolic Velocity} - \text{End Diastolic Velocity}}{\text{Peak Systolic Velocity}}$$

The presence of an arteriovenous fistula increases velocities in the arteries leading to the fistula and may exceed levels associated with stenosis.

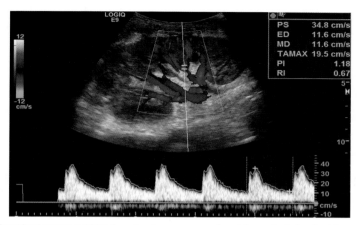

Superficial vessels and high flow give clear sonograms from intrarenal arteries. Resistance index and pulsatility index are in the normal range.

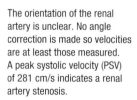

The orientation of the renal artery is unclear. No angle correction is made so velocities are at least those measured. A peak systolic velocity (PSV) of 281 cm/s indicates a renal artery stenosis.

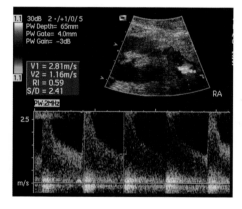

FURTHER READING

Baxter GM, Ireland H, Moss JG, Harden PN, Junor BJR, Rodger RSC. Colour Doppler ultrasound in renal transplant artery stenosis: Which Doppler index? *Clin Radiol*. 1995; 50:618–622.

Cochlin DLL, Wake A, Salaman JR, Griffin PJA. Ultrasound changes in the transplant kidney. *Clin Radiol*. 1988; 39:373–376.

Dodd GD, Tublin ME, Shah A, Zajko AB. Imaging of vascular complications associated with renal transplants. *AJR Am J Roentgenol*. 1991; 157:449–459.

Pancreas transplantation

PREPARATION
None.

POSITION
Supine or right anterior oblique position.

TRANSDUCER
2.0–6.0 MHz curvilinear transducer.

METHOD
Often the entire pancreas is transplanted with a section of duodenum anastomosed to the bladder. The gland is situated in the pelvis, with the venous anastomosis between the donor portal vein and the anterior aspect of the recipient external or common iliac vein. The arterial anastomosis is from the recipient anterior wall of the common iliac artery to a patch of donor aorta containing the celiac trunk and superior mesenteric artery.

APPEARANCE
Uniform pattern of reflectivity similar to that of muscle. Rejection appears as gland enlargement, focal or diffuse areas of low reflectivity, and a resistance index (RI) of > 0.7 (measured in the donor arterial trunk). Imaging is paramount in the follow-up of a pancreatic transplant as clinical and biochemical evaluation is relatively insensitive in determining episodes of acute rejection. Ultrasound evaluation and guidance will allow percutaneous biopsy to confirm the diagnosis and institute therapy. Pancreatic duct exocrine drainage is via the bladder.

MEASUREMENTS
Size of normal gland

	Anteroposterior dimension
Head	3 cm
Body	2.5 cm
Tail	2.5 cm
Pancreatic duct	≤ 3 mm

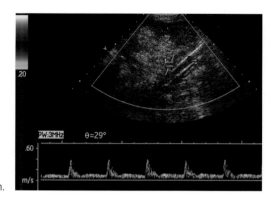

Color Doppler is used to locate the main graft vessels and demonstrate patency, and the RI may be calculated from the arterial spectral waveform.

Color Doppler should be used to locate and show the patency of the main graft artery and vein. RI of the artery should be ≤ 0.7.

FURTHER READING

Heller MT, Bhargava P. Imaging in pancreatic transplants. *Indian J Radiol Imaging*. 2014; 24:339–49.

Morelli L, Di Candio G, Campatelli A, Vistoli F, Del Chiaro M, Balzano E, Croce C, Moretto C, Signori S, Boggi U, Mosca F. Role of color Doppler sonography in post-transplant surveillance of vascular complications involving pancreatic allografts. *J Ultrasound*. 2008; 11:18–21.

Nikolaidis P, Amin RS, Hwang CM, McCarthy RM, Clark JH, Gruber SA, Chen PC. Role of sonography in pancreatic transplantation. *Radiographics*. 2003; 23:939–49.

4

GENITAL TRACT

Venus Hedayati, Dean Y. Huang,
Keshthra Satchithananda, and
Paul S. Sidhu (Male Genital Tract);
Induni Douglas, Anthony E. Swartz,
and Wui K. Chong (Female Genital
Tract)

MALE GENITAL TRACT

Testes

PREPARATION
None.

POSITION
Supine, with towel beneath the scrotum to provide support.

TRANSDUCER
7.0–13.0 MHz linear transducer.

METHOD
Compare reflectivity between the two sides on a single image. Obtain transverse and longitudinal images.

APPEARANCE
The testes are homogenous and of medium level reflectivity. The mediastinum testis is a highly reflective linear structure in the posterior-superior aspect of the testicle draining the seminiferous tubules of the testes into the rete testis. Drainage from here is via the epididymis to the seminal vesicles. The rete testis is a low-reflective area at the hilum of the testis with finger-like projections into the parenchyma. Apart from these projections, the parenchyma of the testis should remain of homogenous reflectivity. The appendix testis is present in the majority of patients, most commonly at the superior testicular pole or in the groove between the testis and the head of the epididymis medially. There is marked variation in its size and appearance; it is usually oval, although a stalk-like structure is occasionally seen.

MEASUREMENTS
Scrotal wall thickness ranges from 2–8 mm, depending on cremasteric muscular contraction.

Average testis size is length 3.8 cm (3.5–5.5 cm) × width 3.0 cm (2.1–4.0 cm) × height 2.5 cm (1.5–2.5 cm).

Testis volume measurement is calculated using the formula:

$$\text{Length} \times \text{Width} \times \text{Height} \times 0.71.$$

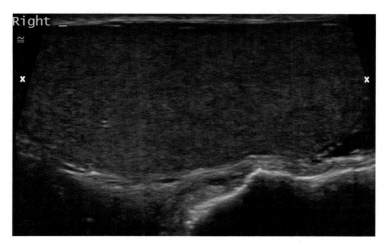

A longitudinal view with the length measurement (between cursors) demonstrating homogenous medium-level echogenicity.

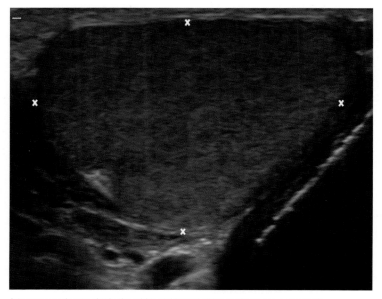

A transverse view to obtain the width and height of the testis (between cursors).

A prepubescent volume is 1–2 ml and at puberty volume is > 4 ml.

Average volume is 18.6 ± 4.8 ml. A total volume (both testis) of > 30 ml is indicative of normal function. A testis volume < 12 ml is associated with lower testicular function.

Testicular volume greater than 2 ml allows reliable appreciation of intra-testicular color Doppler flow.

Small veins drain from the mediastinum testis to the pampiniform plexus. A varicocele is present if the veins measure > 2 mm.

FURTHER READING

Arai T, Kitahara S, Horiuchi S, Sumi S, Yoshida K. Relationship of testicular volume to semen profiles and serum hormone concentrations in infertile Japanese males. *Int J Fertil*. 1998; 43:40–47.

Hricak H, Filly RA. Sonography of the scrotum. *Invest Radiol*. 1983;18:112–121.

Ingram S, Hollman AS. Colour Doppler sonography of the normal paediatric testis. *Clin Radiol*. 1994; 49:266–267.

Kim W, Rosen MA, Langer JE, Banner MP, Siegelman ES, Ramchandani P. US MR imaging correlation in pathologic conditions of the scrotum. *Radiographics*. 27: 1239–1253.

Leung ML, Gooding GAW, Williams RD. High-resolution sonography of scrotal contents in asymptomatic subjects. *AJR Am J Roentgenol*. 1984; 143:161–164.

Paltiel HJ, Diamond DA, Di Canzio J, Zurakowski D, Borer JG, Atala A. Testicular volume: Comparison of orchidometer and US measurements in dogs. *Radiology*. 2002; 222:114–119.

Sakamoto H, Saito K, Oohta M, Inoue K, Ogawa Y, Yoshida H. Testicular volume measurement: Comparison of ultrasonography, orchidometry, and water displacement. *Urology*. 2007; 69:1:152–157.

Epididymis

PREPARATION
None.

POSITION
Supine, with towel beneath the scrotum to provide support.

TRANSDUCER
7.0–13.0 MHz linear transducer.

METHOD
Transverse and longitudinal images, to include the head, body, and tail.

APPEARANCE
- The **head** (globus major) is a pyramid-shaped structure lying superior to the upper pole of the testis. It is of iso- or hyperreflectivity to the testis with a coarser echotexture.
- The **body** courses along the posterolateral aspect of the testicle. The echotexture and reflectivity often render it inseparable from the surrounding peritesticular tissue.
- The **tail** (globus minor) is slightly thicker than the body and can be seen as a curved structure at the inferior aspect of the testicle where it becomes the proximal portion of the ductus deferens.

The appendix epididymis is not as frequently seen as the appendix testis. It projects from the epididymis from different sites, most commonly the head. It usually has a stalk-like appearance.

MEASUREMENTS
The epididymis is 6–7 cm in length.
- The **head** measures 5–12 mm maximal length and 10–12 mm in diameter.
- The **body** measures 2–4 mm (average 1–2 mm) in diameter.
- The **tail** measures 2–5 mm.

FURTHER READING
Krone KD, Carroll BA. Scrotal ultrasound. *Radiologic Clin North Am.* 1985; 23:121–139.

Leung ML, Gooding GAW, Williams RD. High-resolution sonography of scrotal contents in asymptomatic subjects. *AJR Am J Roentgenol.* 1984; 143:161–164.

Oyen RH. Scrotal ultrasound. *Eur Radiol.* 2002; 12:19–34.

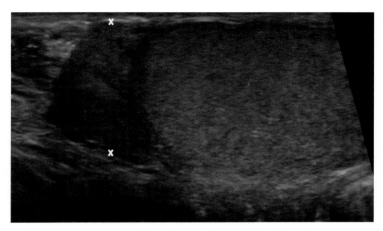

A longitudinal view of the head of the epididymis (between cursors).

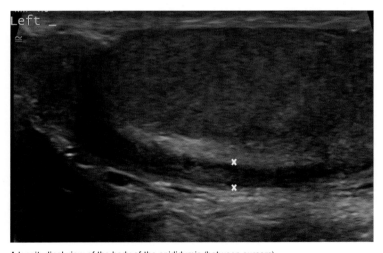

A longitudinal view of the body of the epididymis (between cursors).

Varicoceles

PREPARATION
None.

POSITION
Supine, with towel beneath the scrotum to provide support.

TRANSDUCER
7.0–13.0 MHz linear transducer.

METHOD
The patient should ideally be imaged supine during and following the Valsalva maneuver and then the process should be repeated with the patient standing. The diameter of the veins should be measured in B-Mode.

Incidence:
- Left-sided varicoceles are more common (80%) as the right testicular vein drains directly and obliquely into the IVC.
- Bilateral varicocele: 15%
- Isolated right-sided: varicocele: 5%

The varicocele may be primary (incompetent/absent valves in the testicular vein) or secondary (increased intravenous pressure due to compression, e.g., renal vein thrombus, renal carcinoma, or portal hypertension). A renal sonographic examination is suggested when a varicocele, particularly an isolated right-sided varicocele, is demonstrated to exclude a secondary cause, but this remains controversial.

Intratesticular varicoceles are much rarer (< 2% symptomatic population) than extratesticular varicoceles (< 20% of general population; 40% of subfertile or infertile men). They are usually found at the mediastinum testis, and when present they are often found in association with an ipsilateral extratesticular varicocele. Left-sided intratesticular varicoceles are more common.

APPEARANCE
Small veins drain from the mediastinum testis to the pampiniform plexus. A varicocele is present if the veins measure > 2–3 mm.

They will have a characteristic serpiginous appearance and vascular flow. Flow reversal may be seen with the Valsalva maneuver.

Grading of varicocele with Doppler ultrasound

Grade	Findings
1	No dilated intrascrotal veins Reflux in spermatic cord veins of the inguinal channel during Valsalva maneuver
2	Small posterior varicosities that extend to the superior pole of the testis Increase in diameter and reflux flow at upper pole (supratesticular) during Valsalva maneuver
3	No major dilatation in supine position Dilated veins at the lower (inferior) pole of testis seen on standing Reflux at lower pole during Valsalva maneuver
4	Dilated veins seen in supine position and more marked in an upright position and during Valsalva maneuver Reflux during Valsalva maneuver
5	Dilated veins, even in prone decubitus position Reflux without Valsalva maneuver and does not increase during Valsalva maneuver

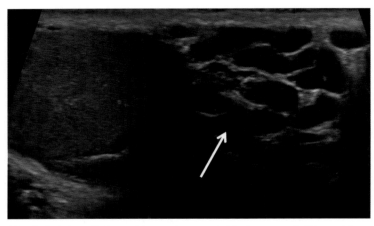

A longitudinal view with the serpiginous veins present at the lower aspect of the scrotal sac (arrow).

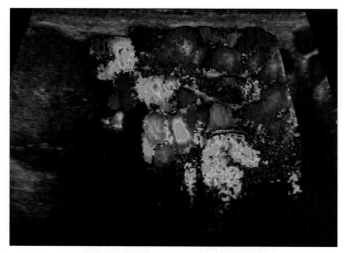

A longitudinal view with the serpiginous veins present at the lower aspect of the scrotal sac distending and demonstrating reflux with the Valsalva maneuver.

FURTHER READING

Das KM, Prasad K, Szmigielski W, Noorani N. Intratesticular varicocele: Evaluation using conventional and Doppler sonography. *AJR Am J Roentgenol.* 1999; 173: 1079–1083.

El-Saeity NS, Sidhu PS. Scrotal varicocele, exclude a renal tumour. Is this evidence based? *Clin Radiol.* 2006; 61:593–599.

Pauroso S, DiLeo N, Fulle I, DiSegni M, Alessi S, Maggini E. Varicocele: Ultrasonographic assessment in daily practice. *J Ultrasound.* 2011; 14:199–204.

Sarteschi LM. Lo studio del varicocele con eco-color-Doppler. *G Ital Ultrasonologia.* 1993; 4:43–49.

Prostate (transrectal sonography)

PREPARATION
None.

POSITION
Left lateral.

TRANSDUCER
A dedicated transrectal transducer is used, which may vary in frequency from 5.0–9.0 MHz. Single or multiplane transducers may be used.

METHOD
The examination is best performed with the patient's bladder half full to provide a contrast to the high-reflective perivesicular fat surrounding the prostate. Axial and longitudinal images can be obtained.

APPEARANCE
The prostate is usefully separated into a peripheral zone and a central gland (encompassing the transition and central zones, and periurethral glandular area). The peripheral zone encompasses 70% of the glandular tissue and appears as medium-level uniform low reflectivity, separated from the central gland by the surgical capsule, which is often of high reflectivity.

MEASUREMENTS
Measurement of the anteroposterior (H), transverse (W), and cephalocaudal (L) dimensions, with the volume calculated, is made by using the formula:

$$\text{Volume} = \pi/6 \times W^2 \times H \times L \ (\pi/6 = 0.524)$$

The normal prostate measures 2.5–3.0 × 2.5–3.0 × 2.0–2.5 cm with an estimated volume of 20–30 ml *but is dependent on age.*

FURTHER READING

Eri LM, Thomassen H, Brennhovd B, Haheim LL. Accuracy and repeatability of prostate volume measurements by transrectal ultrasound. *Prostate Cancer Prostate Dis.* 2002; 5:273–278.

Terris MK, Stamey TA. Determination of prostate volume by transrectal ultrasound. *J Urol.* 1991; 145:984–987.

Villers A, Terris MK, McNeal JE, Stamey TA. Ultrasound anatomy of the prostate: The normal gland and anatomical variations. *J Urol.* 1990; 143:732–738.

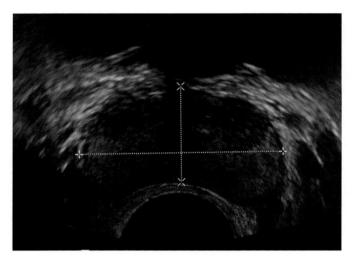

Anteroposterior and transverse measurements of the prostate (between cursors).

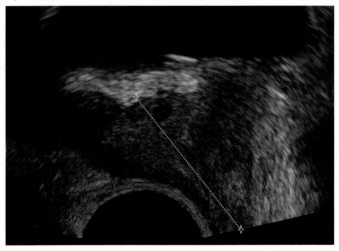

Cephalo-caudal measurement of the prostate (between cursors).

Seminal vesicles (transrectal sonography)

PREPARATION
None.

POSITION
Left lateral.

TRANSDUCER
A dedicated transrectal transducer, which may vary in frequency from 5.0–9.0 MHz, is used. Single or multiplane transducers may be used.

METHOD
The examination is best performed with the patient's bladder half full to provide a contrast to the high-reflective perivesicular fat surrounding the seminal vesicles. Axial and longitudinal images can be obtained.

APPEARANCE
The seminal vesicles are seen as flat-paired structures lying behind the bladder, posterior to and above the base of the prostate gland. The center of the gland is of low reflectivity, with areas of high reflectivity corresponding to the folds of the excretory epithelium; the vas deferens joins with the midline seminal vesicle to make the ejaculatory duct, which enters at the verumontanum. If distended, the wall appears to be composed of two layers. The vas deferens bilaterally can be identified behind the bladder as they run inward and posteriorly to become the ampulla. The junction of the seminal vesicle with the ejaculatory duct usually lies well within the prostate. The ejaculatory complex from each side lies in a communal muscular envelope, which can be identified; the actual lumen of the normal ejaculatory ducts is not normally visible.

MEASUREMENTS
The size of the seminal vesicles varies with age, and comparative assessment of each side in an individual subject may be of more value than to the general population. They range from 2–4 cm in long axis, with an average volume of 13.7 ml.

Measurement of the anteroposterior, transverse, and cephalo-caudal dimensions, with the volume calculated, is made by using the formula:

$$\frac{\text{Anteroposterior Dimension} \times \text{Transverse Dimension} \times \text{Cephalo-caudal Dimension}}{0.5}$$

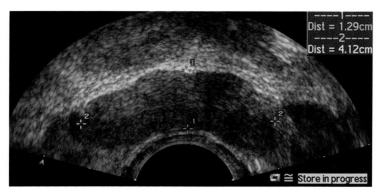

Cephalo-caudal measurement of the prostate seminal vesicle (between cursors).

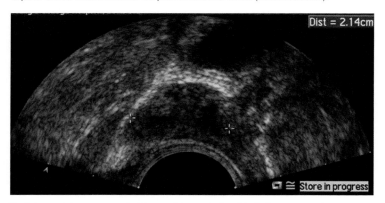

Cephalo-caudal measurement of the prostate seminal vesicle (between cursors).

Age range	Bilateral volume
20–29 years	9.3 ± 3.9 ml
30–39 years	9.7 ± 1.3 ml
40–49 years	10.1 ± 2.6 ml
50–59 years	9.3 ± 2.4 ml
60–69 years	7.5 ± 1.7 ml
70–79 years	6.1 ± 4.5 ml
80–89 years	5.1 ± 1.1 ml

FURTHER READING

Carter SSC, Shinohara K, Lipshultz LI. Transrectal ultrasonography in disorders of the seminal vesicles and ejaculatory ducts. *Urol Clin North Am.* 1989; 16:773–789.

Terasaki T, Watanabe H, Kamoi K, Naya Y. Seminal vesicle parameters at 10-year intervals measured by transrectal ultrasonography. *J Urol.* 1993; 150:914–916.

Penis

PREPARATION
None.

POSITION
Patient is supine, and the penis is examined on the dorsal aspect.

TRANSDUCER
7.5–10.0 MHz linear transducer.

APPEARANCE
The body of the penis consists of two paired corpora cavernosa and the corpus spongiosum (containing the urethra), which lies on the ventral surface of the fused corpora cavernosa. The cavernosal artery and the dorsal artery supply the penis. Color and spectral Doppler ultrasound, with the addition of a pharmacological stimulant to produce an erection, allows for the assessment of arterial flow disorders as well as of venous leakage in erectile dysfunction.

METHOD
The penis is imaged longitudinally and horizontally in the flaccid state to detect areas of fibrosis and calcification to indicate Peyronie's disease. A baseline assessment of the spectral Doppler waveform of the right cavernosal artery, as close to the base of the penis as possible (the peno-scrotal junction), should be attempted to achieve the optimal angle of insonation (< 60°) and to reduce the effect of distal arterial variants. The baseline peak systolic velocity (PSV) in a longitudinal plane is recorded. Following the intracavernosal injection of 20 micrograms Prostaglandin E1 (PGE1), measurements of the PSV and end-diastolic velocity (EDV) are made every 5 minutes for 20–25 minutes at the same level in the right cavernosal artery. If a sub-optimal response to pharmacological stimulation is identified, administration of the intracavernosal alpha-adrenergic antagonist phentolamine (2 mg), which blocks the increased sympathetic drive in the anxious patient, may supplement the examination.

MEASUREMENTS
Increased systolic and diastolic flow early in tumescence, which decreases with eventual reversed diastolic flow as veno-occlusion occurs, would be expected following pharmaco-stimulation in a normal study. A guide to differentiation among arteriogenic, venogenic,

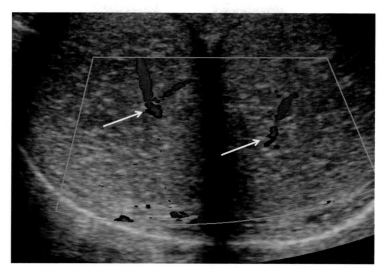

A transverse image through the paired corpora cavernosum, with the paired central cavernosal arteries (arrows) present centrally. The right or left cavernosal artery is targeted in a longitudinal view to measure the velocity.

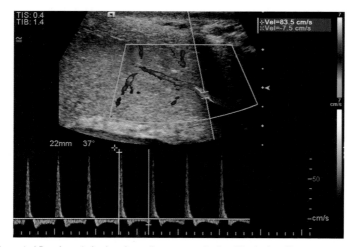

A spectral Doppler gate is placed over the cavernosal artery 20 minutes after pharmacostimulation with the spectral Doppler waveform indicating a normal response; elevation of the peak systolic velocity and reversal of diastolic flow.

and nonvascular dysfunction assessed 25 minutes after cavernous stimulation with 20 micrograms PGE1 is illustrated in the following table:

Type of dysfunction	Peak systolic velocity	End diastolic velocity
Arterial insufficiency	< 25 cm/sec	—
Venogenic impotence	> 35 cm/sec	> 5 cm/sec
Normal values	> 25 cm/sec	< 5 cm/sec

FURTHER READING

Andresen R, Wegner HEH. Assessment of the penile vascular system with color-coded duplex sonography and pharmacocavernosometry and -graphy in impotent men. *Acta Radiologica*. 1997; 38:303–308.

Benson CB, Aruny JE, Vickers MA. Correlation of duplex sonography with arteriography in patients with erectile dysfunction. *AJR Am J Roentgenol*. 1993; 160:71–73.

Halls J, Bydawell G, Patel U. Erectile dysfunction: The role of penile Doppler ultrasound in diagnosis. *Abdominal Imaging*. 2009; 34:712–725.

Quam JP, King BF, James EM, Lewis RW, Brakke DM, Ilstrup DM, Parulkar BG, Hattery RR. Duplex and color sonographic evaluation of vasculogenic impotence. *AJR Am J Roentgenol*. 1989; 153:1141–1147.

Wilkins CJ, Sriprasad S, Sidhu PS. Colour Doppler ultrasound of the penis. *Clin Radiol*. 2003; 58:514–523.

FEMALE GENITAL TRACT

Ovarian volume (transvaginal sonography)

PREPARATION
Empty bladder prior to the examination.

POSITION
Lithotomy position on adapted examination couch.

TRANSDUCER
8.4 MHz curved transvaginal transducer.

METHOD
The longest diameter of the ovary is obtained (d1).

Maximum anteroposterior diameter (d2) is obtained perpendicular to d1.

The transducer is then rotated 90°, and d3 is measured perpendicular to d2.

$$\text{Ovarian volume} = d1 \times d2 \times d3 \times 0.523 \text{cm}^3$$

APPEARANCE
Ovoid structure between the uterus and muscular pelvic sidewall. The internal iliac vessels are posterior to the ovaries. The presence of follicles is the hallmark of their identification. These could be multiple developing follicles, one or more dominant follicles, or a corpus luteum. The postmenopausal ovary is small and homogenous in echo-texture.

MEASUREMENT
$$\text{Ovarian volume} = d1 \times d2 \times d3 \times 0.523 \text{cm}^3$$

Age (years)	Mean volume (cm³) ± SD
< 30	6.6 ± 0.19
30–39	6.1 ± 0.06
40–49	4.8 ± 0.03
50–59	2.6 ± 0.01
60–69	2.1 ± 0.01
> 70	1.8 ± 0.01

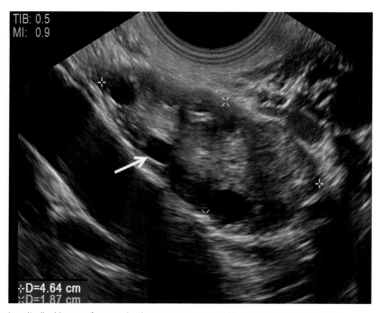

Longitudinal image of a reproductive age group ovary with measurements d1 and d2.
A follicle (arrow) is the hallmark of a reproductive ovary.

Mean ovarian volume of reproductive age group women: 4.9 ± 0.03 cm³ (upper limit 20 cm³)

Mean ovarian volume of postmenopausal women: 2.2 ± 0.01 cm³ (upper limit 10 cm³)

FURTHER READING

Bruchim I, Aviram R, Halevy RS, Beyth Y, Tepper R. Contribution of sonographic measurement of ovarian volume to diagnosing ovarian tumors in postmenopausal women. *J Clin Ultrasound.* 2004; 2:107–114.

Pavlik EJ, DePriest PD, Gallion HH, Ueland FR, Reedy MB, Kryscio RJ, van Nagell JR Jr. Ovarian volume related to age. *Gynecol Oncol.* 2001; 80:333–334.

Ovarian follicles (transvaginal sonography)

PREPARATION
Empty bladder prior to the examination.

POSITION
Lithotomy position on adapted examination couch.

TRANSDUCER
8.4 MHz curved transvaginal transducer.

METHOD
Maximum diameter of follicle is obtained.

APPEARANCE
Ovarian follicles are thin and smooth walled, round or oval, anechoic spaces in ovaries, without flow by means of color Doppler ultrasound.

Corpus luteum is a cyst with diffusely thick walls and crenulated inner margins with a ring of vascularity at the periphery. Hemorrhage may result in internal echoes within the corpus luteum, without internal flow on color Doppler.

MEASUREMENT

Reproductive age group	Maximum diameter
Dominant follicle	3 cm*
Nondominant follicle	1.4 cm
Corpus luteum	3 cm*

*Maximum diameter of a dominant follicle and a corpus luteum cyst is taken as 3 cm but according to the Society of Radiologists in Ultrasound criteria 2010, simple ovarian cysts are also taken as almost certainly benign and do not need follow-up in this age group.

Maximum number of follicles per ovary should be < 12 in reproductive age group.

Postmenopausal age group	Maximum diameter
Ovarian cyst	1 cm

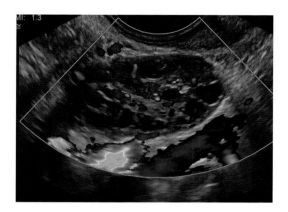

Multiple follicles in a
reproductive ovary.

FURTHER READING

Levine D, Brown DL, Andreotti RF, Benacerraf B, Benson CB,
Brewster WR, Coleman B, DePriest P, Doubilet PM, Goldstein
SR, Hamper UM, Hecht JL, Horrow M, Hur HC, Marnach
M, Patel MD, Platt LD, Puscheck E, Smith-Bindman R.
Management of asymptomatic ovarian and other adnexal cysts
imaged at US: Society of Radiologists in Ultrasound consensus
conference statement. *Ultrasound Quarterly*. 2010; 26:121–131.
Rotterdam E. SHRE/ASRM-Sponsored PCOS Consensus Workshop
Group Revised 2003 consensus on diagnostic criteria and long-
term health risks related to polycystic ovary syndrome. *Fertil.
Steril.* 2004; 81:19–25.

Uterus (transvaginal sonography)

PREPARATION
Empty bladder prior to the examination.

POSITION
Lithotomy position on adapted examination couch.

TRANSDUCER
8.4 MHz curved transvaginal transducer.

METHOD
Mid-sagittal section of the uterus is taken. The total uterine length (L) is measured from the top of the fundus to the external cervical os. The maximum anterior-posterior (AP) diameter is measured perpendicular to the maximum L. The transducer is then rotated 90° to obtain maximum transverse (TRV) diameter in a transverse section.

APPEARANCE
Uniform pattern of medium-strength echoes with a highly reflective central stripe called the endometrial stripe.

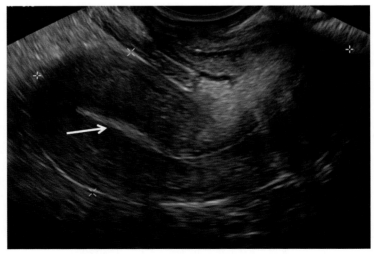

Mid-sagittal section of the uterus. The endometrial stripe is seen as a highly reflective stripe (arrow) and the cursors indicate the uterine length (L) and anteroposterior (AP) diameter.

MEASUREMENT

Age	Mean length (L)	Mean anteroposterior (AP)	Mean width (TRV)
Reproductive age group			
Nulliparous (P = 0)	7.3 cm	3.2 cm	4.0 cm
Primiparous (P = 1)	8.3 cm	3.9 cm	4.6 cm
Multiparous (P > = 2)	9.2 cm	4.3 cm	5.1 cm
Postmenopausal			
Early(< 5 years)	6.7 cm	3.1 cm	3.6 cm
Late (> 5 years)	5.6 cm	2.5 cm	3.1 cm

FURTHER READING

Merz E, Miric-Tesanic D, Bahlmann F, Weber G, Wellek S. Sonographic size of uterus and ovaries in pre- and postmenopausal women. *Ultrasound Obst Gynaecol.* 1996; 7:38–42.

Platt JF, Bree RL, Davidson D. Ultrasound of the normal non-gravid uterus: Correlation with gross and histopathology. *J Clin Ultrasound.* 1990; 18:15–19.

Endometrial stripe thickness (transvaginal sonography)

PREPARATION
Empty bladder prior to the examination.

POSITION
Lithotomy position on adapted examination couch.

TRANSDUCER
8.4 MHz curved transvaginal transducer.

METHOD
Endometrial thickness is taken in the sagittal plane of the uterus at the thickest part near the fundus, including both endometrial layers, from basal layer of the anterior wall to the basal layer of the posterior uterine wall, excluding any intracavitatory fluid.

APPEARANCE
During menstruation: The endometrium appears as a thin echogenic line.

Proliferative phase (days 6–14): The endometrium becomes thicker and more echogenic relative to the myometrium, reflecting the development of glands, blood vessels, and stroma.

Late proliferative (periovulatory) phase: The endometrium develops a multilayered appearance with an echogenic basal layer and hypoechoic inner functional layer, separated by a thin echogenic median layer arising from the central interface or luminal content.

Secretory phase: The endometrium becomes even thicker and more echogenic. It reaches a maximum thickness during the mid-secretory phase.

Postmenopausal: The endometrium appears thin, homogeneous, and echogenic.

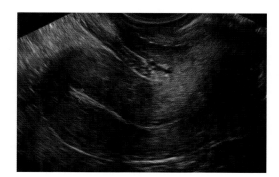

During the proliferative phase, the endometrium (between cursors) measures 6 mm.

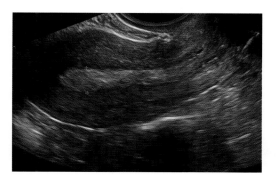

During the secretory phase, the endometrium (between cursors) measures 16 mm.

MEASUREMENT

Age group		Maximum thickness (range, mean ± 2 SD)
Reproductive age group		
Phase of cycle	Menstrual	4 mm (1–4 mm)
	Proliferative	7 mm (mean 7.63 ± 3.82 mm)
	Secretory	16 mm (mean 8.65 ± 4.21 mm)
Postmenopausal	Symptomatic	4 mm
	Asymptomatic	5 mm

Focal heterogeneity or eccentric thickening of the endometrium detected should always be further investigated irrespective of endometrial thickness.

The value of endometrial thickness in reproductive age group women is less important because it may vary widely depending on the phase of the menstrual cycle. The examination should ideally be performed during the early proliferative phase (day 6–10) of the menstrual cycle, after the endometrium has sloughed.

Imaging should be performed on a postmenopausal woman on hormonal replacement, at the beginning or end of a cycle of treatment, when the endometrium is at its thinnest as any pathologic thickening will be more prominent at this stage.

FURTHER READING

Bennett GL, Andreotti RF, Lee SI, Dejesus Allison SO, Brown DL, Dubinsky T, Glanc P, Mitchell DG, Podrasky AE, Shipp TD, Siegel CL, Wong-You-Cheong JJ, Zelop CM. ACR appropriateness criteria (R) on abnormal vaginal bleeding. *J Am Coll Radiol.* 2011; 8:460–468.

Nalaboff KM, Pellerito JS, Ben-Levi E. Imaging the endometrium: Disease and normal variants. *Radiographics.* 2001; 21:1409–1424.

Ozdemir S, Celik C, Gezginc K, Kiresi D, Esen H. Evaluation of endometrial thickness with transvaginal ultrasonography and histopathology in premenopausal women with abnormal vaginal bleeding. *Arch Gynecol Obstet.* 2010; 282:395–399.

Saatli B, Yildirim N, Olgan S, Koyuncuoglu M, Emekci O, Saygili U. The role of endometrial thickness for detecting endometrial pathologies in asymptomatic postmenopausal women. *Aust NZ J Obstet Gynaecol.* 2014; 54:36–40.

5

GASTROINTESTINAL TRACT

Anu E. Obaro and Suzanne M. Ryan

Appendix

PREPARATION
Full bladder. After a 10-minute search for the appendix on full bladder, if the search is negative, ask the patient to empty the bladder and continue the search.

POSITION
Supine and left lateral decubitus position if retrocecal appendix is suspected.

TRANSDUCER
5.0–10.0 MHz linear array transducer or a 3.0–7.0 MHz curvilinear transducer.

METHOD
Place transducer transversely below the edge of the right hepatic lobe, in front of the right kidney, and slowly move down to the right iliac fossa along the line of the ascending colon. Identify the cecum and then trace the appendix; it is draped over the right iliac vessels anterior to the iliopsoas muscle.

APPEARANCE
Features of a normal appendix include:
1. A compressible blind-ended tubular structure
2. Surrounded by normal-appearing fat
3. Wall thickness < 3 mm, measured from the serosa to the lumen, and diameter measurement of < 6 mm, measured from serosa to serosa.

Caution: In normal appendices nonexpressible inspissated feces may result in an outer diameter > 6 mm; therefore, mural thickness is a more sensitive indicator of inflammation.

MEASUREMENTS
Typically, appendicitis is characterized by a wall thickness > 3 mm and a diameter > 6 mm. Since a maximal diameter > 6 mm may be seen in the absence of appendicitis, the following must also be considered: intraluminal content, periappendiceal change, hypervascular mural flow with color Doppler, or loss of wall layers.

Variation in age is only marginally significant. Acute appendicitis in the pediatric population is diagnosed if the appendiceal diameter is > 5.7 mm and wall thickness is > 2.2 mm.

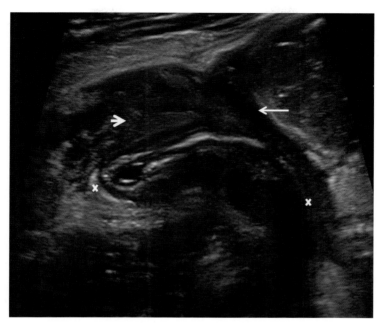

The tubular structure (between cursors) is the inflamed appendix with free fluid (arrow). Note the presence of inflamed increased hyperechoic fat (arrowhead), so that the appendix "stands out."

FURTHER READING

Je BK, Kim SB, Lee SH, Lee KY, Cha SH. Diagnostic value of maximal-outer-diameter and maximal-mural-thickness in use of ultrasound for acute appendicitis in children. *World J Gastroenterol.* 2009; 15: 2900–2903.

Park NH, Park CS, Lee EJ, Kim MS, Ryu JA, Bae JM, Song JS. Ultrasonographic findings identifying the fecal-impacted appendix: Differential findings with acute appendicitis. *Br J Radiol.* 2007; 80: 872–877.

Simonovský V. Normal appendix: Is there any significant difference in the maximal mural thickness at US between pediatric and adult populations? *Radiology.* 2002; 224:333–337.

Simonovsky V. Sonographic detection of normal and abnormal appendix. *Clin Rad.* 1999; 54; 533–539.

Upper gastrointestinal tract wall (endoscopic ultrasound)*

PREPARATION
The patient is sedated and given pharyngeal local anesthesia.

POSITION
Left lateral position.

TRANSDUCER
An ultrasonic endoscope consisting of a 7.5 MHz ultrasound mechanical sector-scan transducer housed in an oil-filled chamber at the tip of a specially adapted fiber-optic endoscope.

METHOD
After introduction of the endoscope to the desired position under direct vision, intraluminal gas is aspirated.

Three methods are available for exploration of the upper GI tract wall:
1. Direct apposition of the transducer on the mucosa: used for the esophagus.
2. Contact of a small balloon filled with water over the tip of the ultrasonic transducer: used for the esophagus, and gastric and duodenal walls.
3. Direct instillation of deaerated water, usually about 500 ml: for gastric and duodenal walls.

APPEARANCE
The ultrasound beam passing through the gastrointestinal wall will potentially encounter six interfaces between tissue layers, which allow the visualization of five separate layers. These layers have their respective histological correlates.

*This is a specialized procedure and is conducted in a similar manner to standard upper gastrointestinal endoscopy.

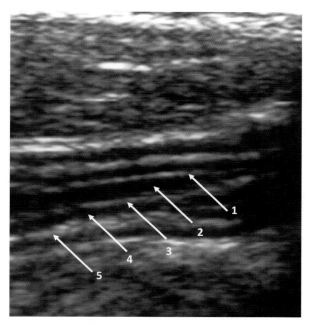

The gastrointestinal wall is visualized as six interfaces between tissue layers, which result in the depiction of five separate layers: layer 1, luminal/mucosa; layer 2, deep mucosa; layer 3, submucosa; layer 4, muscularis propria; layer 5, adventitia/serosa.

Layer 1	High reflective line	Luminal/mucosa
Layer 2	Low reflectivity	Deep mucosa
Layer 3	High reflectivity	Submucosa
Layer 4	Low reflectivity	Muscularis propria
Layer 5	High reflectivity	Adventitia/serosa

MEASUREMENT

The accuracy of endoscopic ultrasound measurements is affected by physiological peristalsis, with a wide variation in normal wall thickness. Measurements are also affected by interobserver variability, differences in the frequency of transducer, and differences in pressure application. Esophageal wall thickness is 2.4 mm in normal controls, which is statistically lower than in patients with a histological grade of Barrett's esophagus.

FURTHER READING

Dietrich CF. Esophagus, stomach, duodenum. In: *Endoscopic Ultrasound: An Introductory Manual and Atlas*. Stuttgart: Thieme, 2011: Chapter 13.

Gill KR, Ghabril MS, Jamil LH, Al-Haddad M, Gross SA, Achem SR, Woodward TA, Wallace MB, Raimondo M, Hemminger LL, Wolfsen HC. Variation in Barrett's esophageal wall thickness: Is it associated with histology or segment length? *J Clin Gastroenterol*. 2010; 44:411–415.

Shorvon PJ, Lees WR, Frost RA, Cotton PB. Upper gastrointestinal endoscopic ultrasonography in gastroenterology. *Br J Radiol*. 1987; 60:429–438.

Gastrointestinal tract wall (transabdominal ultrasound)

PREPARATION

None (reference values are applicable regardless of fasting state).

POSITION

Supine.

TRANSDUCER

7.0–12.0 MHz linear transducer.

METHOD

Bowel wall thickness may be measured before and after ingestion of 480 ml of water. Measurements should be made only on images obtained in transverse sections. In the nondistended state, bowel segments demonstrate a target configuration. The thickness of the bowel wall is measured from the edge of the high-reflective core representing the intraluminal gas and mucus, to the low-reflective outer border representing the bowel wall. In the distended state (following ingestion of water), the lumen is fluid filled. Distension is considered adequate when the luminal diameter is greater than 8 cm for the stomach, 3 cm for the small bowel, and 5 cm for the large bowel. Measurements should be made from the low-reflective intraluminal fluid to the interface representing the serosa.

APPEARANCE

The gastrointestinal (GI) tract has a layered appearance on ultrasound as described previously, and these five layers are evident when using frequencies of 5 MHz or more. Although it has been shown that thickness of the bowel wall depends on the amount of distension, patient weight, and patient age, pathological thickening should be suspected when it measures more than 2 mm (except in gastric antrum, duodenum, and rectum).

MEASUREMENT

GI wall tract thickness is dependent on transducer frequency, patient weight, and patient age.

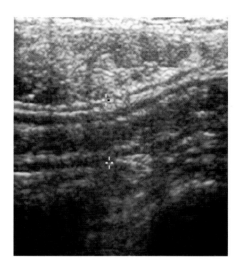

Normal transverse colon (between cursors) with no fecal residue present.

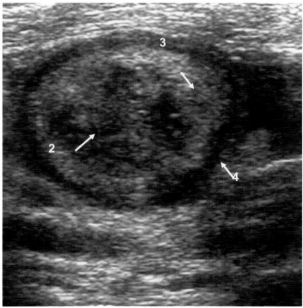

Transverse image not at an absolute right angle (layers 1 and 5 not visualized), demonstrating layer 2, deep mucosa; layer 3, submucosa; and layer 4, muscularis propria.

GI tract wall thickness (mm) according to transducer frequency

Location	Frequency	
	8 MHz	12 MHz
Gastric antrum	3.1 ± 0.8	2.9 ± 0.8
Duodenum	1.6 ± 0.3	1.6 ± 0.3
Jejunum	0.9 ± 0.2	0.9 ± 0.2
Ileum	1.2 ± 0.3	1.1 ± 0.3
Colon	1.0 ± 0.2	1.0 ± 0.3
Sigmoid colon	1.2 ± 0.3	1.2 ± 0.3
Rectum	2.1 ± 0.5 (4 MHz transducer)	

FURTHER READING

Fleischer AC, Muhletaler CA, James AE Jr. Sonographic assessment of the bowel wall. *AJR Am J Roentgenol.* 1981; 136:887–891.

Nylund K, Hausken T, Odegaard S, Eide GE, Gilja OH. Gastrointestinal wall thickness measured with transabdominal ultrasonography and its relationship to demographic factors in healthy subjects. *Ultraschall Med.* 2012; 33:E225–232.

Anal endosonography

PREPARATION
None.

POSITION
Left lateral position. Females should be examined prone due to the symmetry of the anterior perineal structures in this position.

TRANSDUCER
A high-frequency (7–10 MHz) rotating rectal transducer is used, which provides a 360° image. A hard sonolucent plastic cone covers the transducer and is filled with degassed water for acoustic coupling. The cone is covered with a condom with ultrasound gel applied to both surfaces.

METHOD
Serial images are obtained on slow withdrawal of the transducer down the anal canal. Images are typically taken at the upper, mid, and lower anal canal.

APPEARANCE
The normal anal canal is composed of five distinct layers: mucosa, submucosa, internal anal sphincter, intersphincteric plane, and external anal sphincter.

Mucosa: This low-reflective layer is immediately adjacent to the transducer and is continuous with the rectal mucosa.

Submucosa: This high-reflective layer lies between the mucosa and the internal anal sphincter, becoming progressively thicker and denser caudally.

Internal anal sphincter: The smooth muscle of the internal sphincter is seen as a homogeneous low reflective circular band > 2–3 mm in width, extending caudally to a level just proximal to the anal verge. The thickness should be measured at the 3 o'clock or 9 o'clock positions.

Intersphincteric: This is a narrow high-reflective band between the two sphincter planes.

External anal sphincter (EAS): The striated muscle of the external anal sphincter has mixed reflectivity and a linear pattern giving a "streaky" appearance. The EAS can be traced from the puborectalis component of the levator ani muscle to its cutaneous termination. The EAS is consistent in appearance for both sexes posterolaterally. However, anteriorly, in females, the muscle is deficient in the immediate region of the perineal body and vagina. In males, the sphincter tapers anteriorly into two arcs that meet in the midline.

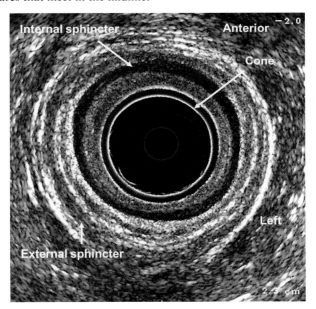

View taken at the mid anal canal level demonstrating the internal sphincter (measuring 3 mm) and the striated appearance of the external sphincter.

MEASUREMENTS

| | Average thickness (mm) | |
	Female	Male
Internal sphincter (increases with age*)	1.8–3.8	1.9–3.4
External sphincter	4.0–7.7	6.1–8.6
Longitudinal muscle	2.5–2.9	2.3–2.9

*0.38 mm every 10 years

FURTHER READING

Abdool Z, Sultan AH, Thakar R. Ultrasound imaging of the anal sphincter complex: A review. *Br J Radiol.* 2012; 85:865–75.

Beets-Tan RG, Morren GL, Beets GL, Kessels AG, el Naggar K, Lemaire E, Baeten CG, van Engelshoven JM. Measurement of anal sphincter muscles: Endoanal US, endoanal MR imaging, or phased-array MR imaging? A study with healthy volunteers. *Radiology.* 2001; 220:81–89.

Law PJ, Bartram CI. Anal endosonography: Technique and normal anatomy. *Gastrointest Radiol.* 1989; 14:349–353.

Sultan AH, Kamm MA, Hudson CN, Nicholls JR, Bartram CI. Endosonography of the anal sphincters: Normal anatomy and comparison with manometry. *Clin Radiol.* 1994; 49:368–374.

6 SUPERFICIAL STRUCTURES

Keshthra Satchithananda and
Paul S. Sidhu

Parathyroid glands

PREPARATION
None.

POSITION
Supine.

TRANSDUCER
7.0–14.0 MHz linear transducer.

METHOD
Images are obtained in the longitudinal and transverse planes.

APPEARANCE
The four normal parathyroid glands are generally located at the poles of the thyroid lobes, although the inferior parathyroid glands may be ectopic, found in the upper mediastinum. Occasionally, the normal parathyroid gland can be identified separate from thyroid tissue, especially in a longitudinal view. A linear high-reflective band representing an aponeurosis or a fibrous sheath may surround the gland. The normal parathyroid gland may either be seen as a slightly low-reflective or slightly high-reflective oval area adjacent to the normal thyroid. A parathyroid adenoma is identified as an oval-shaped, low-reflective area, with increased color Doppler flow, in the expected location of a parathyroid gland.

MEASUREMENTS
The average normal parathyroid measures 5 × 3 × 1 mm but is difficult to image. The enlarged parathyroid adenoma is normally visible as an oval-shaped, low-reflective area adjacent to the thyroid gland, most often located at the inferior aspect of the left thyroid lobe.

FURTHER READING
Reeder SB, Desser TS, Weigel RJ, Jeffrey RB. Sonography in primary hyperparathyroidism. Review with emphasis on scanning technique. *J Ultrasound Med.* 2002; 21:539–552.

Simeone JF, Mueller PR, Ferrucci JT Jr., van Sonnenberg E, Wang CA, Hall DA, Wittenberg J. High-resolution real-time sonography of the parathyroid. *Radiology.* 1981; 141:745–751.

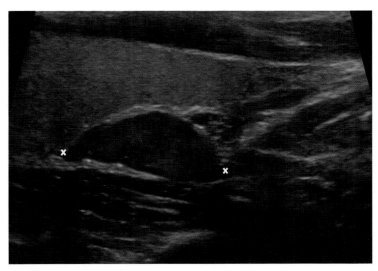

Longitudinal view demonstrating the oval hyporeflective parathyroid adenoma (between cursors), surrounded by the hyperreflective aponeurosis.

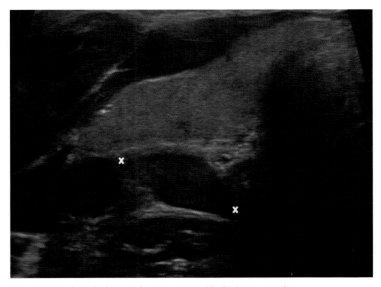

The same parathyroid adenoma (between cursors) in the transverse view.

Submandibular salivary glands

PREPARATION
None.

POSITION
Supine.

TRANSDUCER
7.0–14.0 MHz linear array transducer.

METHOD
The gland is imaged in two planes: paramandibular and frontal.

APPEARANCE
Homogenous high-reflective parenchyma, well demarcated from the surrounding tissues.

MEASUREMENTS
Three measurements are obtained: anteroposterior and lateral-medial direction, and then depth.

Volume is calculated as if the gland is a spherical body with the formula:

$$\text{Volume} = \frac{\pi \times \text{height} \times (\text{diameter})^2}{4}$$

	Normal values
Anteroposterior length	35 ± 5.7 mm
Paramandibular length (depth)	14.3 ± 2.9 mm
Lateral-medial length	33.7 ± 5.4 mm

FURTHER READING
Dost P, Kaiser S. Ultrasonographic biometry in salivary glands. *Ultrasound Med Biol.* 1997; 23:1299–1303.

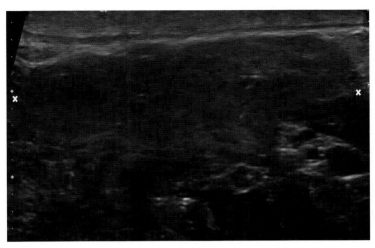

The submandibular gland in a paramandibular view, to measure the lateral-medial length.

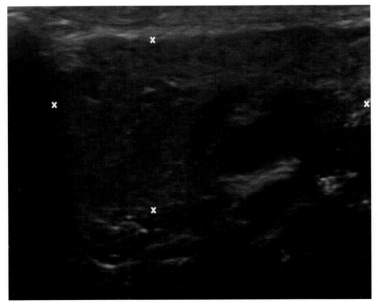

The submandibular gland in a longitudinal view, to measure the anteroposterior and depth measurements.

Parotid salivary glands

PREPARATION
None.

POSITION
Supine.

TRANSDUCER
7.0–14.0 MHz linear array transducer.

METHOD
The gland is imaged in a transverse plane and in an axis parallel to the ramus of the mandible (parallel direction to the normal dental occlusion).

APPEARANCE
The gland is homogeneous and of high reflectivity, more so than that of the submandibular gland.

MEASUREMENTS

Axis parallel to ramus of mandible	46.3 ± 7.7 mm
Dimension in transverse axis	37.4 ± 5.6 mm
Parotid parenchyma:	
Lateral to mandible	7.4 ± 1.7 mm
Dorsal to mandible	22.8 ± 3.6 mm

FURTHER READING
Dost P, Kaiser S. Ultrasonographic biometry in salivary glands. *Ultrasound Med Biol.* 1997; 23:1299–1303.

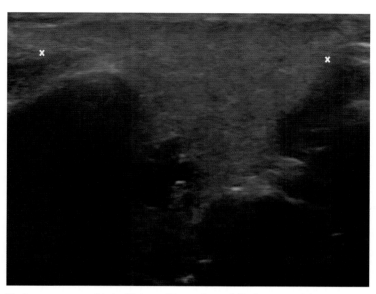

The homogenous parotid gland is imaged in an axis parallel to the ramus of the mandible, in the direction of the dental occlusion.

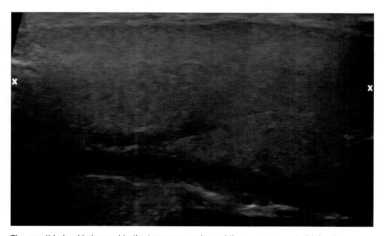

The parotid gland is imaged in the transverse axis, and the measurement obtained.

Thyroid gland

PREPARATION
None.

POSITION
Supine with the neck extended.

TRANSDUCER
7.0–14.0 MHz linear transducer.

METHOD
Longitudinal and transverse images obtained in the lower half of the neck from the midline.

APPEARANCE
Below the subcutaneous tissues is a 1–2 mm thin, low-reflective line corresponding to the platysma muscle. Anterior to this is a thin, high-reflective line representing the superficial cervical aponeurosis. The thyroid gland is made up of two lobes connected medially by the isthmus, which has a transverse course. Approximately 10%–40% of normal people have a third lobe (pyramidal) arising from the isthmus that runs upward along the same longitudinal axis as the thyroid lobes but lies in front of the thyroid cartilage. The thyroid parenchyma has a fine homogeneous echo pattern, which is of higher reflectivity than the contiguous muscular structures and is interrupted at the periphery by the arterial and venous vessels.

MEASUREMENTS

Age	Length	Anteroposterior diameter
Newborn	18–20 mm	8–9 mm
1 year	25 mm	12–15 mm
Adult	40–60 mm	13–18 mm

The mean thickness of the isthmus is 4–6 mm.

Thyroid volume may be calculated using the right and left anteroposterior lobe measurements and the following formula:

$$\text{Volume} = [6.91 \times \text{RAP}] + [3.05 \times \text{LAP}] - 3.48$$

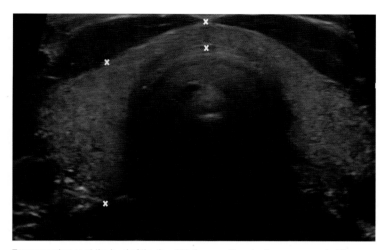

Transverse image at the level of the thyroid isthmus, with a depth measurement of the isthmus, and a depth measurement of the right lobe.

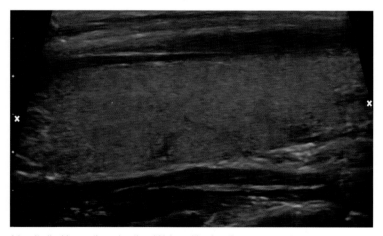

A longitudinal image through a thyroid lobe, with a length measurement.

The difference in thyroid volume between males and females is explained solely by a difference in body weight.

Male thyroid volume is 19.6 ± 4.7 ml; female is 17.5 ± 3.2 ml.

Doppler studies of the thyroid arteries: There are two thyroid arteries on each side, superior and inferior. Rarely, a third artery is present in the midline and is named the arteria ima.

- Mean diameter of these vessels is 1–2 mm.
- Peak systolic velocity is 20–40 cm/second.
- End diastolic velocity is 10–15 cm/second.

The thyroid veins originate from the perithyroid venous plexus and join to form three main groups, which drain into the ipsilateral jugular vein. The largest vessel is a lower vein and can measure up to 7–8 mm.

FURTHER READING

Hegedus L, Perrild H, Poulsen LR, Andersen JR, Holm B, Schnohr P, Jensen G, Hansen JM. The determination of thyroid volume by ultrasound and its relationship to body weight, age and sex in normal subjects. *J Clin Endocrinol Metabol*. 1983; 56:260–263.

Udea D. Normal volume of the thyroid gland in children. *J Clin Ultrasound*. 1990; 18:455–462.

Vade A, Gottschalk ME, Yetter EM, Subbaiah P. Sonographic measurements of the neonatal thyroid gland. *J Ultrasound Med*. 1997; 16:395–399.

Lymph nodes in the neck

PREPARATION
None.

POSITION
Supine.

TRANSDUCER
7.0–14.0 MHz linear transducer.

METHOD
Use the thyroid as a landmark and assess the anterior and posterior aspects of both aspects of the neck.

APPEARANCE
Ultrasound features that should be assessed include:

1. **Lymph node shape:** Assessed by measuring the longitudinal (L) and transverse (T) diameter on the same image and calculating the L/T ratio. This is normal when L/T > 2; that is, when the shape is oval. Another method is to measure the ratio of the minimum to maximum diameter of a node in the transverse plane. A ratio of more than 0.55 yields the highest accuracy when predicting malignancy with ultrasound.
2. **Nodal hilus:** This should be of high reflectivity and wide. The presence of hilar narrowing or cortical widening (either concentrically or eccentrically) should be regarded with suspicion for malignancy.
3. **Nodal size:** Ultrasound is not a reliable criterion for differentiating benign from malignant lymph nodes.
4. **Calcification:** Calcification is found in a significantly lower number of malignant nodes.
5. **Doppler waveforms:** The Resistance Index can be measured, with a cutoff of 0.70 for differentiating benign (< 0.70) from malignant, but with considerable overlap in recordings.

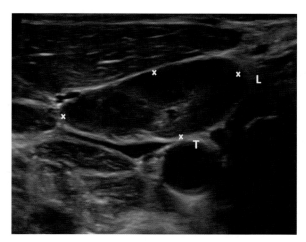

Longitudinal image through an oval lymph node demonstrating features of benign disease. Longitudinal (L) and transverse (T) diameter on the same image, calculating the L/T ratio.

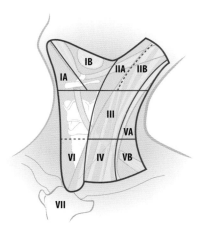

Level classification of lymph nodes of the neck.

MEASUREMENT

Classification of position of neck lymph nodes

Level	Lymph node group	Ultrasound boundaries
IA	Submental	Between anterior bellies of diagastric muscle
IB	Submandibular	Posterior to diagastric muscle below mandible
II	Upper jugular	Skull base to inferior border of hyoid bone
		A: anterior to spinal accessory nerve
		B: posterior to spinal accessory nerve
III	Middle jugular	Inferior border of hyoid to inferior border of cricoid cartilage
IV	Lower jugular	Inferior border of cricoid cartilage to clavicle
V	Posterior triangle	Superior boundary is the convergence of the sternomastoid and trapezius muscles to the clavicle
		A: Above the plane of the inferior cricoid cartilage
		B: Below the plane of the inferior cricoid cartilage
VI	Anterior compartment	Superior boundary hyoid bone to suprasternal notch
VII	Superior mediastinum	Between carotid arteries at the top of manubrium superiorly to innominate vein inferiorly

FURTHER READING

Na DG, Lim HK, Byun HS, Kim HD, Ko YH, Baek JH.
    Differential diagnosis of cervical lymphadenopathy: Usefulness of color Doppler sonography. *AJR Am J Roentgenol*. 1997;
    168:1311–1316.

Robbins KT, Shaha AR, Medina JE, Califano JA, Wolf GT, Ferlito A, Som PM, Day TA. Consensus statement on the classification and terminology of neck dissection. *Arch Otolaryngol Head Neck Surg.* 2008; 134:536–538.

Takashima S, Sone S, Nomura N, Tomiyama N, Kobyashi T, Nakamura H. Nonpalpable lymph nodes of the neck: Assessment with US and US-guided fine needle aspiration biopsy. *J Clin Ultrasound.* 1997; 25:283–292.

Vassallo P, Wernecke K, Roos N, Peters PE. Differentiation of benign from malignant superficial lymphadenopathy: The role of high resolution US. *Radiology.* 1992; 183:215–220.

Orbits (extraocular muscles)

PREPARATION
None.

POSITION
Supine in a reclining position with the eyelid closed.

TRANSDUCER
10.0–14.0 MHz linear transducer.

METHOD
Transverse and longitudinal planes of the four recti are obtained and appear as low-reflective areas.

APPEARANCE
Well-circumscribed, round, low-reflective fluid-like structure, with linear structures posteriorly located corresponding to the intraocular muscles.

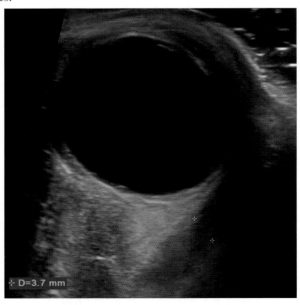

Axial image through the orbit, demonstrating the diameter of the medial rectus muscle (between cursors).

MEASUREMENTS

Diameters of extraocular muscles in normal population

Muscle	Mean (mm)	SD (mm)	Median (mm)
Superior rectus	5.3	0.7	5.4
Lateral rectus	3.0	0.4	3.1
Inferior rectus	2.6	0.5	2.6
Medial rectus	3.5	0.6	3.6

FURTHER READING

Byrne SF, Gendron EK, Glaser JS, Feuer W, Atta H. Diameter of normal extraocular recti muscles with echography. *Am J Opthalmol.* 1991; 112:706–713.

Orbits (optic nerve)

PREPARATION
None.

POSITION
Supine in a reclining position, with eyelid closed.

TRANSDUCER
10.0–14.0 MHz linear transducer.

APPEARANCE
Tubular structure. Homogenous, low-reflective, parallel nerve fiber bundle surrounded by a highly reflective dural sheath.

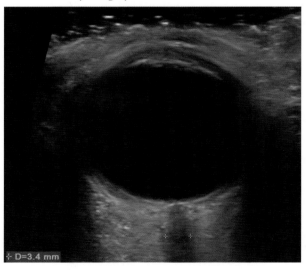

Axial image through the orbit demonstrating the optic nerve (between cursors).

MEASUREMENTS
Optic nerve width: 2.4 mm–3.4 mm

Median of 2.9 mm and no more than 0.3 mm between the two nerves.

FURTHER READING
Atta HR. Imaging of the optic nerve with standardized echography. *Eye*. 1988; 2:358–366.

7

PERIPHERAL VASCULAR (ARTERIAL)

*Colin R. Deane and
Paul S. Sidhu*

Upper limbs (peripheral arteries)

PREPARATION
Patient should rest in a supine position. If accurate physiological changes are to be measured, then the subject should rest for 15 minutes in a room where the temperature is 21°C to avoid vasoconstriction.

POSITION
Supine.

TRANSDUCER
3.0–10.0 MHz linear transducer for subclavian and axillary arteries, higher frequency (8.0–15.0 MHz) linear transducer for brachial, radial, and ulnar arteries.

METHOD
Examination of the upper extremity usually starts at the level of the subclavian artery followed by the axillary artery, brachial artery, and radial and ulnar arteries. The radial and ulnar arteries are imaged with the arm in supination, and slightly abducted. The vessels should be examined in the longitudinal axis.

APPEARANCE
The arteries appear as noncompressible, pulsating tubular structures. At rest, flow waveforms show a high peripheral resistance spectral Doppler waveform with a typical tri- (or greater) phasic flow pattern, consisting of a steep systolic upslope, a systolic peak, a reverse flow component, forward flow in late diastole, and pre-systolic zero. The flow waveform is dependent on environmental factors and changes markedly if the hand is subjected to cold or heat.

Arterial disease. Arms suffer less from atherosclerotic disease than do legs. Occlusions, for example from thrombus or injury, are evident as absent flow in arteries with damped flow distally. Stenoses or arterial compression are evident as local increases in velocity with damped flow distally if the disease is severe.

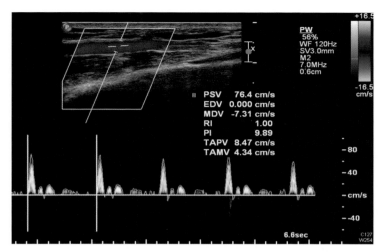

Radial artery flow waveform at rest. The flow waveform shows high-resistance pulsatile flow.

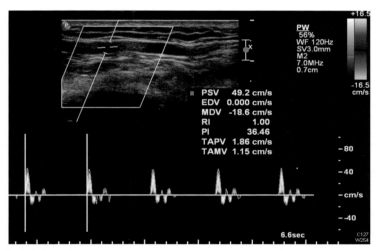

With the hand placed in cold water, velocities are reduced and there is increased reverse flow indicating distal vasoconstriction.

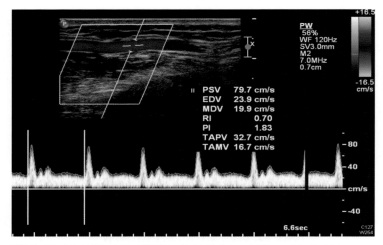

With the hand placed in warm water, there is greatly increased flow, evident in higher mean velocities and reduced pulsatility and resistance indices.

MEASUREMENTS
As in subclavian artery, Peak Systolic Velocity = 100 ± 49 cm/s.

Artery	Diameter (mm ± SD)	Peak systolic velocity (cm/sec ± SD)
Brachial	3.5 ± 0.9	75 ± 18
Radial (wrist)	2.8 ± 0.6	57 ± 16
Ulnar (wrist)	2.8 ± 0.6	66 ± 27

FURTHER READING
Trager S, Pignataro M, Anderson J, Kleinert JM. Color flow Doppler: Imaging the upper extremity. *J Hand Surg (Am)*. 1993; 18:621–625.

Abdominal aorta and common iliac arteries

PREPARATION
None.

POSITION
Supine.

TRANSDUCER
1.0–5.0 MHz curvilinear transducer.

APPEARANCE
Pulsating tubular low-reflective structure lying slightly to the left of the midline, anterior to the vertebral column. The distal aorta is most often involved in aneurysmal dilatations. Arteries are aneurysmal if there is a 50% focal increase in diameter.

METHOD
The patient's arms are along the body to relax the abdominal wall.

The aorta is imaged in longitudinal from a sagittal, coronal, and oblique axis and also in transverse to understand its shape and course. Diameter measurements in the beam direction are most reliable where the vessel wall is most clearly defined.

Diameter measurements should be made in long section from coronal and sagittal view. In the case of aneurysms, these views show the point of maximum diameter clearly. Transverse views may overestimate aneurysm diameter if the aorta axis is significantly curved.

When aligned to the ultrasound beam, the artery wall appears as a bright line. Measurements have been reported from the inner walls of the aorta and from the outer walls. Outer-to-outer wall diameter is typically 2–2.5 mm greater than the inner-to-inner measurement. It is important to state which measurement has been made.

The common iliac artery diameter is measured just distal to the aortic bifurcation or at its largest diameter. Images are obtained in transverse and longitudinal views; diameter is measured in long sections for reasons described above.

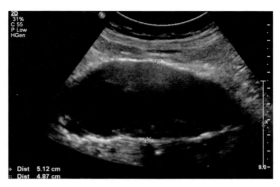

Longitudinal measurement of aortic aneurysm. The diameter based on calipers placed on the outer to outer edges of the aneurysm wall is 2.5 mm greater than that measured from its inner edges.

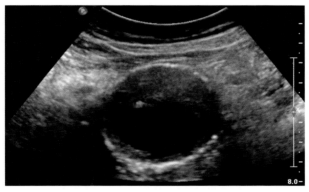

Transverse image of an aortic aneurysm. The anterior-posterior view gives clear definition of the artery wall. The lateral edges are less clearly defined.

MEASUREMENTS

The following measurements are inner-to-inner wall measurements. The locations are:

- **Proximal diameter:** At the level of the confluence of the splenic and portal veins and the left renal vein.
- **Distal diameter:** Measure just above the aortic bifurcation.

Proximal aorta	Vessel diameter (Mean ± SD) mm	Range (mm)
15–49 years		
Male	16.9 ± 2.4	12–22
Female	15.0 ± 2.4	11–22
50–89 years		
Male	19.9 ± 3.4	14–28
Female	18.3 ± 2.7	14–25
Distal aorta	Vessel diameter (Mean ± SD) mm	Range (mm)
15–49 years		
Male	15.1 ± 1.7	12–19
Female	12.7 ± 1.3	10–16
50–89 years		
Male	16.8 ± 2.9	11–23
Female	14.6 ± 1.9	11–18
Common iliac artery	Vessel diameter (Mean ± SD) mm	Range (mm)
15–49 years		
Male	9.7 ± 1.2	7.5–11.5
Female	8.5 ± 1.0	6–10
50–89 years		
Male	10.1 ± 2.0	6.5–16.5
Female	9.2 ± 1.3	7–13

FURTHER READING

Johnston KW, Rutherford RB, Tilson MD, Shah DM, Hollier L, Stanley JC. Suggested standards for reporting on arterial aneurysms. Subcommittee on Reporting Standards for Arterial Aneurysms, Ad Hoc Committee on Reporting Standards,

Society for Vascular Surgery and North American Chapter, International Society for Cardiovascular Surgery. *J Vas Surg.* 1991; 13:452–458.

Pedersen OM, Aslaksen A, Vik-Mo H. Ultrasound measurement of the luminal diameter of the abdominal aorta and iliac arteries in patients without vascular disease. *J Vas Surg.* 1993; 17:596–601.

Lower limbs (peripheral arteries)

PREPARATION
None.

POSITION
Supine. For the popliteal region and lower leg, the patient should be moved to a lateral decubitus position or the prone position.

TRANSDUCER
Iliac arteries: 1.0–5.0 MHz curvilinear array. Femoral, popliteal, and tibial arteries: typically, a 3.0–8.0 MHz linear transducer. A curvilinear array is also useful for imaging the femoral arteries in large patients.

METHOD
Arteries should be imaged in the longitudinal plane. Color Doppler imaging is used to help identify the course of the arteries, particularly the iliac and proximal tibial arteries. Color flow scale is set to show aliasing at locations of increased velocities. Pulsed spectral Doppler measurements are made with an angle preferably ≤ 60°.

APPEARANCE
The arteries appear as noncompressible, pulsating tubular structures. In the presence of severe calcification, color and spectral Doppler interrogation is difficult. At rest the Doppler waveforms show a typical triphasic flow waveform. Color flow at rest shows rapid changes in the cardiac cycle.

MEASUREMENTS
Common femoral artery diameters have been shown to increase with age and are larger in men than women.

Velocities in peripheral arterial disease
Peripheral artery stenosis grading is usually measured as a velocity ratio comparing the in-stenosis peak velocity to that in the pre-stenosis undiseased vessel. Velocity ratios of 1.8 to 2.8 (the latter for aorto-iliac arteries) have been proposed as diagnostic of 50% stenosis, although a ratio of 2.0 is most commonly used. Higher velocity ratios are indicative of higher grade stenosis.

As an approximate guide, velocity ratios are indicative of the percentage narrowing, absolute velocities more indicative of the hemodynamic effect of a specific stenosis. In stenosis peak velocities have been shown

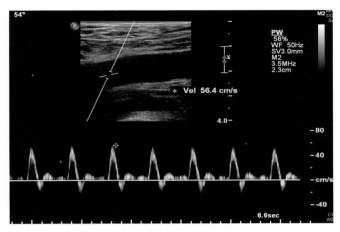

Pulsatile triphasic flow in a healthy common femoral artery at rest.

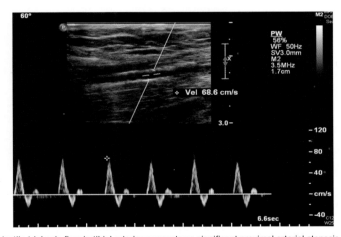

Pulsatile triphasic flow in tibial arteries suggests no significant proximal arterial stenosis.

to have correlation with pressure gradient through iliac artery stenosis. Flow waveforms are useful to indicate the presence of proximal disease. As the stenosis or occlusion becomes more severe, pulsatility of the downstream flow waveform is reduced.

Color flow imaging shows aliasing at the site of a stenosis. The spectral Doppler shows peak velocities increasing threefold from pre-stenosis to in-stenosis with a maximum PSV of approximately 3.5 m/s, indicative of a significant stenosis.

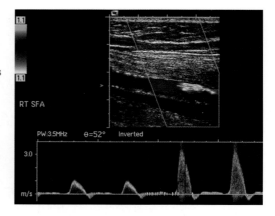

Damped monophasic flow in an anterior tibial artery is indicative of severe proximal arterial disease.

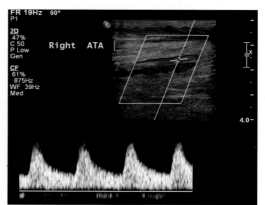

Aneurysms

Arterial aneurysms are usually described as such if there is a 50% increase in arterial diameter. Popliteal artery diameters of greater than 10 mm are aneurysmal.

Normal artery diameter and resting peak systolic velocities (average of proximal and distal) are listed in the following table:

Artery	Diameter ± SD (cm)	PSV ± SD (cm/s)
External iliac	0.79 ± 0.13	98 ± 17.5*
Common femoral	0.82 ± 0.14	80 ± 16*
Proximal superficial femoral	0.6 ± 0.12	73 ± 10
Distal superficial femoral	0.54 ± 0.11	56 ± 12
Deep femoral	–	64 ± 15
Popliteal	0.52 ± 0.11	53 ± 17*
Distal anterior tibial	–	56 ± 20
Distal posterior tibial	–	48 ± 23
Distal peroneal	–	44 ± 12

*Average of proximal and distal.

FURTHER READING

Hatsukami TS, Primozich J, Zierler RE, Strandness DE Jr. Color Doppler characteristics in normal lower extremity arteries. *Ultrasound Med Biol.* 1992; 18:167–171.

Jager KA, Ricketts HJ, Strandess DE. Duplex scanning for the evaluation of lower limb arterial disease. In Bernstein EF, ed. *Noninvasive Diagnostic Techniques in Vascular Disease.* St. Louis: Mosby, 1985.

Legemate DA, Teeuwen, C, Hoeneveld H, Eikelboom BC. How can the assessment of the hemodynamic significance of aorto-iliac arterial stenosis by duplex scanning be improved? A comparative study with intraarterial pressure measurement. *J Vas Surg.* 1993; 17:676–684

Sandgren T, Sonesson B, Ahlgren AR, Lanne T. The diameter of the common femoral artery in healthy human: Influence of sex, age, and body size. *J Vas Surgery.* 1999; 29:503–510.

Strauss AL, Roth FJ, Rieger H. Noninvasive assessment of pressure gradients across iliac artery stenoses: Duplex and catheter correlative study. *J Ultrasound Med.* 1993; 12:17–22.

Wolf YG, Kobzantsev Z, Zelmanovich L. Size of normal and aneurysmal popliteal arteries: A duplex ultrasound study. *J Vas Surg.* 2006; 43:488–492.

Lower limbs (peripheral artery bypass grafts)

PREPARATION
None.

POSITION
Supine. For the popliteal region and lower leg, the patient should be moved to a later decubitus position or the prone position.

TRANSDUCERS
Iliac arteries and grafts: 1.0–5.0 MHz curvilinear array. Femoral, popliteal, and tibial arteries, typically 3.0–8.0 MHz linear transducer. A curvilinear array is also useful for the femoral arteries in large patients.

METHOD
The arteries and graft should be imaged in the longitudinal plane. Color Doppler imaging is used to help identify the course of the arteries and graft, particularly the iliac and proximal tibial arteries. Color flow scale is set to show aliasing at locations of increased velocities. Pulsed spectral Doppler measurements are made with an angle preferably ≤ 60°.

Measurement of ankle brachial pressure indices (ABI) of the limb is also recommended. These can reveal progression of inflow or outflow arterial disease as well as stenosis of the graft itself.

APPEARANCE
The arteries appear as noncompressible, pulsating tubular structures. The graft can be synthetic (usually PTFE) or formed from a vein. It is important to establish the level and location of the graft, especially in the early postoperative period when the leg may be swollen and access limited.

MEASUREMENTS
Although absolute velocities have been used to define stenosis level, the variation in graft diameter between patients leads to similar variance in normal velocities, although velocities > 300 cm/s are usually indicative of significant narrowing. The velocity ratio of peak systolic velocity (PSV) in the stenosis to that in an adjacent undiseased segment compensates for variation in diameter and flow. For moderate stenoses, velocity ratios of 1.5 and 2.0 have been proposed. For severe stenoses, velocity ratios of 3.0 and 3.5 are indicative of impending failure. At

Color flow shows a change in velocity. The spectral Doppler sample volume has been moved from pre-stenosis where PSV is low (42 cm/s) to in-stenosis where PSV rises more than tenfold indicating a tight stenosis that is threatening graft patency.

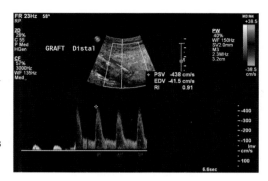

Flow waveform showing staccato-type flow indicating severe downstream stenosis.

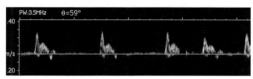

this level of stenosis, a decrease in ankle/brachial pressure index (ABPI) of > 0.15 is evident.

Particular care should be taken when measuring velocity ratios at the distal anastomosis. Size mismatches from the graft to runoff artery can lead to high velocity ratios > 3.0. Careful scanning of the anastomosis and runoff artery can usually establish whether this is a focal stenosis or merely good flow in a narrow artery.

Low velocities in a graft are indicative of inadequate inflow or outflow and suggest early occlusion. A PSV of 45 cm/s, below which velocities should not fall, has been suggested for both vein and PTFE grafts.

Proximal grafts do not require intensive ultrasound surveillance. For infrainguinal grafts a risk stratification table has been proposed with low-risk grafts scanned at 6–12 months.

Category	Maximum PSV (cm/s)	Velocity ratio	Low velocity criterion (cm/s)	ABPI change
Imminent failure (> 70% stenosis with low flow)	> 300	> 3.5	< 45 or staccato graft flow	> 0.15
High risk (> 70% stenosis with normal flow)	> 300	> 3.5	> 45	< 0.15
Moderate risk (50%– 70% stenosis with normal graft flow)	180–300	> 2.0	> 45	< 0.15
Low risk (< 50% stenosis with normal flow)	< 180	< 2.0	> 45	< 0.15

(Table adapted from Tinder et al., 2009)

FURTHER READING

Davies AH, Magee TR, Tennant SWG, Lamont PM, Baird RN, Horrocks M. Criteria for identification of the "at risk" infrainguinal bypass graft. *Eur J Vasc Surg.* 1994; 8:315–319.

Giannoukas AD, Androulakis AE, Labropoulos N, Wolfe JHN. The role of surveillance after infrainguinal bypass grafting. *Eur J Vasc. Endovasc Surg.* 1996; 11:279–289.

Idu MM, Buth J, Cuypers P, Hop WC, van de Parvoordt ED, Tordoir JM. Economising vein-graft surveillance programs. *Eur J Vasc Endovasc Surg.* 1998; 15:432–438.

Tinder CN, Bandyk DF. Detection of imminent vein graft occlusion: What is the Optimal Surveillance Program? *Semin Vasc Surg.* 2009; 22:252–260.

Westerband A, Mills JL, Kistler S, Berman SS, Hunter GC, Marek JM. Prospective validation of threshold criteria for intervention in infrainguinal vein grafts undergoing duplex surveillance. *Ann Vasc Surg.* 1997; 11:44–48.

Hemodialysis access fistulas and grafts

PREPARATION
None.

POSITION
Seated or supine with the couch back raised for patient comfort.

TRANSDUCERS
Low/high-frequency linear array transducer (typically 4.0–9.0 MHz and 7.0–14.0 MHz). Low-frequency transducers allow better imaging of high velocities in the circuit and improved imaging of deep arteries and veins. Superficial transducers provide more detail of the superficial vein or graft. For optimum imaging, two transducers are often needed.

METHOD

Pre-fistula assessment
Arm vessels are assessed to plan the optimum site for fistula or graft. The cephalic and basilic veins are assessed. Minimum diameter is measured and evidence of thrombus and major side branches noted. A tourniquet may be used. The arteries are examined for normal flow, level of brachial artery bifurcation, and radial artery diameter. Central veins are assessed for patency.

Post-fistula/graft surgery
The fistula or graft circuit is investigated to assess access flow and to examine for stenosis, thrombosis, aneurysm, pseudoaneurysm, or other features that may result in inadequate dialysis or problems during dialysis. It is important to ascertain the reason for the examination, for example low flows, and thrombus at the dialysis needling site or high needle pressures, as this may help to focus attention on a specific location in the circuit.

The volume flow is measured in an artery supplying the fistula, either the subclavian, axillary, or proximal brachial artery. Although not all the flow in the artery is to the fistula, this is a more reliable measurement than measuring within the vein where irregular cross-sectional area and turbulence make accurate assessment difficult. For radiocephalic fistulas, measurement should be made in the brachial artery proximal to the radial/ulnar bifurcation since the fistula may be supplied by both arteries.

Volume Flow Measurement = Cross-sectional Area × Mean Velocity

Area can be calculated from the artery diameter. Mean velocity is calculated across one or more cardiac cycles. Potential errors are large from:

- Inaccurate measurement of diameter.
- Erroneous beam/flow "Doppler" angle correction.
- Not insonating the entire artery; the sample volume must encompass the artery width.
- Incorrect Doppler filter setting, allowing either wall or venous signals to reduce mean velocity or removing low-velocity signals from flow near the wall.

It is prudent to make several measurements of volume flow. The circuit is examined from artery to central vein. B-mode and color flow appearances are combined with measurements of peak systolic velocities to assess the circulation.

In cases of suspected steal phenomena, flow waveforms from the radial, ulnar, and distal arteries can be made.

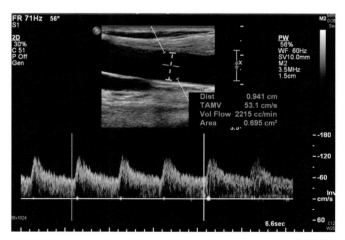

Hemodialysis access volume flow measurement. The sonogram shows pulsatile laminar flow in the brachial artery. A time averaged mean velocity (TAMV) is calculated, which is multiplied by the cross-sectional area based on diameter to give volume flow in the artery supplying the fistula.

MEASUREMENTS

Pre-fistula mapping
Vein diameter should be ≥ 2.0 mm without a tourniquet or ≥ 2.5 mm with a tourniquet. Radial artery diameter should be ≥ 2.0 mm with a triphasic flow waveform.

Post-fistula creation

Volume flow
A large range of flows is possible depending on the site, age, and vessel dimensions. Fistula flows of 500–1200 ml/min are adequate for dialysis, although lower flows are sometimes adequate in radiocephalic fistulas. Flows up to 3,000 ml/min are not unusual; flows over 2,000 ml/min may be associated with cardiac insufficiency. Fistulas tolerate lower flows than do grafts, which have increased risk of thrombosis.

Recommendations for lower flow limits requiring further investigation and intervention are:

European Best Practice Guideline Recommendations

Grafts:	Flow < 600 ml/min or > 20% reduction in flow/month
Forearm fistulas:	Flow < 300 ml/min

National Kidney Foundation/Kidney Disease Outcomes Quality Initiative Guidelines

Grafts:	Flow < 600 ml /min. Flow 1000 ml/min with decrease > 25% over 4 months
Fistulas:	No absolute measure recommended; flows should be considered for individuals. It is noted that levels of < 400 ml/min and 650 ml/min have been proposed.

Velocities
The fistula circuit contains elevated velocities. Peak systolic velocities (PSVs) at the anastomosis can be > 2.5 m/s with normal function. PSVs of 2.5 m/s in the vein have been used to indicate stenosis, but the high flows and irregularity in venous lumen will result in false positives.

Velocity ratios are indicative of narrowing but are common in older fistula veins. Guidelines suggested for investigation are:

PSV ratio > 2.0 in the supplying artery

PSV ratio > 3.0 in the vein

Velocities should be considered alongside other findings, including any reduction in flow and clinical indications to obtain a complete overview of fistula and graft hemodynamics.

FURTHER READING

National Kidney Foundation. NKF-K/DOQI clinical practice guidelines for vascular access: Update 2006. *Am J Kidney Dis.* 2006; 48 (suppl 1):S177–S277.

Older RA, Gizienski TA, Wilkowski MJ, Angle JF, Cote DA. Hemodialysis access stenosis: Early detection with color Doppler US. *Radiology.* 1998; 207:161–164.

Tordoir J, Canaud B, Haage P, Konner K, Basci A, Fouque D, Kooman J, Martin-Malo A, Pedrini L, Pizzarelli F, Tattersall J, Vennegoor M, Wanner C, ter Wee P, Vanholder R. EBPG on vascular access. *Nephrol Dial Transplant.* 2007; 22(suppl 2):ii88–ii117.

Extracranial arteries

PREPARATION
None.

POSITION
Supine. Neck extended and head turned slightly away from the side being examined.

TRANSDUCER
4.0–8.0 MHz linear transducer. A curvilinear probe can be useful in patients with large necks and/or high carotid bifurcations.

METHOD
Examine the common carotid artery (CCA), internal carotid artery (ICA), external carotid artery (ECA), and vertebral arteries in transverse and longitudinal scans. The ICA normally runs lateral or posterolateral to the ECA in its first part, and the extra-cranial ICA does not give off any branches. The vertebral artery may be examined by imaging the CCA in a long view and angling slightly posteriorly. Images of the vertebral artery may be better with the patient's head facing forward. Velocities are obtained from CCA, ICA, ECA, and vertebral arteries using beam steering and beam/flow angle correction of between 40° and 60°.

APPEARANCE

Waveforms
The spectral Doppler waveform of the ICA is low resistance with a high diastolic component in comparison to the ECA, which is of high resistance with a low diastolic component. The waveform of the CCA is usually of low resistance but may appear as a hybrid of those of the ICA and ECA. The waveform of the vertebral artery is of low resistance, similar to that of the ICA but with lower amplitude.

MEASUREMENTS

	Artery diameters (mm)	
	Men	**Women**
CCA	6.52 ± 0.98	6.10 ± 0.8
ICA	5.11 ± 0.87	4.66 ± 0.78

(From Krejza J et al., 2006)

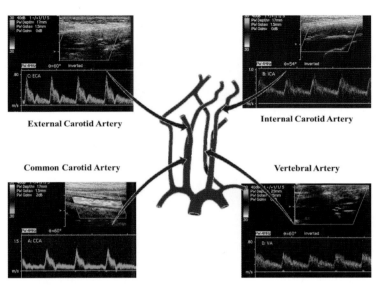

The spectral Doppler waveforms from each of four sites in the extracranial carotid arterial system.

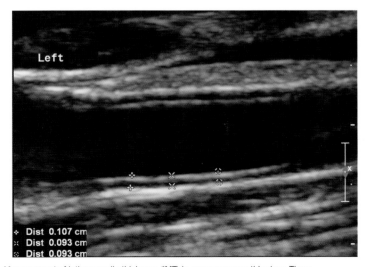

Measurement of intima-media thickness (IMT) in a common carotid artery. Three measurements have been made. The left calipers (+) are not aligned and overestimate the IMT.

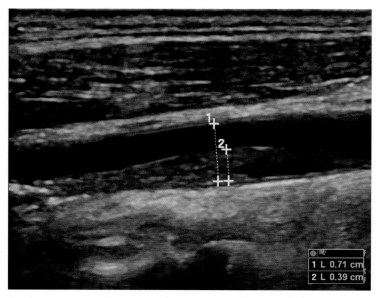

1 L 0.71 cm
2 L 0.39 cm

Clear images of smooth homogeneous plaque allow accurate placement of calipers showing a 55% CCA stenosis.

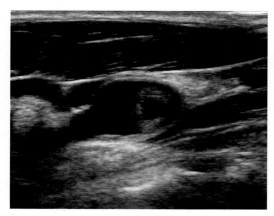

Carotid bulb thrombus. It is important to image the stenosis in a transverse plane to measure the degree of narrowing accurately.

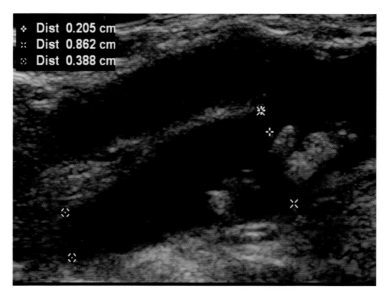

Two measurements of carotid artery stenosis. Based on the bulb diameter at the site of stenosis, the percentage stenosis is 76% (ECST). Based on the patent lumen in the ICA, the percentage stenosis is 47% (NASCET).

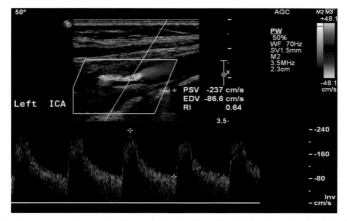

Color flow imaging shows a focal increase in velocities with disturbed flow distally. Pulsed Wave Doppler measurement of peak systolic velocity indicates a 70% stenosis of the ICA.

Plaque/intima-medial thickening
Intima-media thickness is used as an indication of subclinical vascular disease. It differs from plaque, which has been defined as "a focal structure that encroaches into the arterial lumen of at least 0.5 mm or 50% of the surrounding IMT value or demonstrates a thickness of > 1.5 mm as measured from the media-adventitia interface to the intima-lumen interface" (Touboul PJ et al 2007).

Intima-media thickness (IMT)
The inner high-reflective line represents the luminal-intima interface, and the outer high-reflective line represents the media-adventitia interface, with the distance between the two lines being a measure of the thickness of the intima and media combined. Measurements should ideally be taken at several sites and averaged as the mean of the maximum IMT. IMT measurements from the CCA are usually clearer than from the bulb and ICA because of depth and orientation. IMT in the CCA should be measured 1 cm proximal of the bulb. The mean IMT in adults ranges from between 0.5 mm and 1.0 mm with the measurement increasing with age. Values of 1.0 mm or greater are usually taken to be abnormal.

Plaque morphology
B-mode appearance of plaque is described in terms of its:
• Percentage diameter stenosis
• Location
• B-mode ultrasound appearance—plaque texture/morphology
• Surface irregularity

Plaque gray–scale appearance is based on the echogenicity of the plaque. Fatty plaque has low echogenicity, with increasing collagen content leading to higher echogenicity. It has been suggested that fibrous plaques are stable, whereas low-reflectivity plaques are more unstable. Calcification is shown as bright echoes and can cause problems in assessing plaque and lumen patency deep to the calcium. Plaques may also be described as heterogeneous (mixed) or homogenous (uniform). Thrombus may be evident as adhering to the artery wall.

Stenosis criteria
If B-mode images are clear, then these provide the greatest accuracy of stenosis diameter measurement. Two definitions of ICA stenosis are commonly used, arising from European and North American clinical carotid surgery trials. The European (ECST) measurement compares the plaque height as a percentage of the overall diameter of the artery

at the point of maximum stenosis. The North American (NASCET) compares the residual lumen at the stenosis with the lumen of the patient distal ICA. While the latter is a more robust method of measuring stenosis angiographically, it can understate the plaque burden in a carotid bulb (see image on page 165).

Doppler measurements

The CCA peak systolic velocity (PSV) and end diastolic velocity (EDV) are measured in the distal CCA approximately 1 cm proximal to the bulb. Normal ICA PV and EDV are measured just distal to the bulb to avoid the complex hemodynamics within the bulb. At sites of stenosis, the cursor is moved through the stenosis to obtain the maximum velocity.

Normal values

There is a large range of normal PSVs in the ICA, ranging from 20 to 120 cm/s. Velocities are dependent on several factors, including vessel diameter. PSV has been shown to increase significantly with increased systolic blood pressure and pulse pressure and decrease significantly with diastolic blood pressure and age. EDV showed no significant change with systolic, diastolic, or pulse pressure but a significant decrease with age.

Doppler measurement of stenosis

With increased severity of stenosis, B-mode images of plaque become increasingly less clear. Doppler measurement of stenosis has proved effective in determining the level of stenosis of > 50% when PSV shows consistent increases. It does have limitations and errors from physiological causes, anatomical variation, and Doppler instrumentation limitations (e.g., the accuracy of angle correction). Doppler measurements should be assessed alongside the B-mode image and color flow images of the plaque and lumen in long and transverse views.

Higher degrees of stenosis cause higher PSVs until the stenosis becomes so severe that flows and velocities fall, dependent on the severity and length of the stenosis.

The following is based on the NASCET criterion for stenosis. PSV is the main measurement used, although EDV and the ICA/CCA ratio can be helpful.

Percentage stenosis	ICA PSV (cm/s)	ICA/CCA PSV ratio	ICA EDV (cm/s)
< 50	< 125	< 2.0	< 40
50–69	> 125	2.0–4.0	40–100
≥ 70 but less than near occlusion	> 230	> 4.0	> 100
Near occlusion	High or low	Variable	Variable
Occlusion	No flow	N/A	No flow

Vertebral arteries

Vertebral artery flow should be antegrade. There is often asymmetry of artery diameter and flow waveform shape. Systolic hesitation, and partial or full reversal of flow are indicative of incipient or developed subclavian steal.

FURTHER READING

Grant EG, Benson CB, Moneta GL, Alexandrov AV, Baker JD, Bluth EI, Carroll BA, Eliasziw M, Gocke J, Hertzberg BS, Katanick S, Needleman L, Pellerito J, Polak JF, Rholl KS, Wooster DL, Zierler E. Carotid artery stenosis: Gray-scale and Doppler US diagnosis—Society of Radiologists in Ultrasound Consensus Conference. *Radiology.* 2003; 229:340–346.

Krejza J, Arkuszewski M, Kasner SE, Weigele J, Ustymowicz A, Hurst RW, Cucchiara BL, Messe SR. Carotid artery diameter in men and women and the relation to body and neck size. *Stroke.* 2006; 37:1103–1105.

Oates CP, Naylor AR, Hartshorne T, Charles SM, Fail T, Humphries K, Aslam M, Khodabakhsh P. Joint recommendations for reporting carotid ultrasound investigations in the United Kingdom. *Eur J Vasc Endovasc Surg.* 2009; 37:251–261.

Sidhu PS, Allan PL. The extended role of carotid artery ultrasound. *Clin Radiol.* 1997; 52:643–653.

Spencer EB, Sheafor DH, Hertzberg BS, Bowie JD, Nelson RC, Carroll BA, Kliewer MA. Nonstenotic internal carotid arteries: Effects of age and blood pressure at the time of scanning on Doppler US velocity measurements. *Radiology.* 2001; 220:174–178.

Steffen CM, Gray-Weale AC, Byrne KE, Lusby RJ. Carotid atheroma ultrasound appearance in symptomatic and asymptomatic vessels. *Austral N Zealand J Surg.* 1989; 59:529–534.

Touboul PJ, Hennerici MG, Meairs S, Adams H, Amarenco P, Bornstein N, Csiba L, Desvarieux M, Ebrahim S, Fatar M, Hernandez Hernandez R, Jaff, M, Kownator S, Prati P, Rundek T, Sitzer M, Schminke U, Tardi J-C, Taylor A, Vicaut E, Woo KS, Zannad F, Zureik M. Mannheim carotid intima-media thickness consensus (2004–2006). *Cerebrovasc Dis.* 2007; 23:75–80.

Transcranial Doppler (TCD) ultrasound

PREPARATION
None.

POSITION
Patient is supine and facing forward for the transtemporal and trans-orbital views and sitting with the head flexed forward for the transforaminal view.

TRANSDUCER
2.0 MHz phased array.

METHOD

Trans-temporal approach
The cerebral peduncles are identified in the axial/transverse plane in B-mode. Color imaging is used to locate the circle of Willis. The ipsilateral anterior, middle, and posterior cerebral arteries can be identified; flow in the posterior communicating artery may be seen. The contralateral arteries may often be seen. The terminal internal carotid artery may be imaged by tilting the probe down in the axial plane or by viewing in the coronal plane.

Transforaminal approach
Identify the vertebral arteries and follow anteriorly and superiorly to identify the basilar artery.

Transorbital approach
The transducer face is placed on the closed eyelid, directed through the orbit to identify the ipsilateral internal carotid and ophthalmic arteries. Ultrasound output should be kept to maximum mechanical index (MI) of 0.23.

APPEARANCES
Color flow imaging will enable the arteries to be located and aid in the placement of the spectral Doppler gate to measure arterial velocities. The normal spectral Doppler waveforms will reflect the low resistance of the intracranial arteries, with a broad systolic peak and high forward diastolic flow.

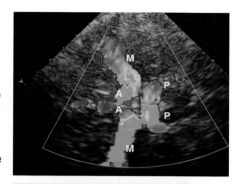

Transtemporal transverse image of the circle of Willis (anterior is to the left of the image). Defocusing through the bone results in poor lateral resolution of the vessels. The R and L MCAs (M), ACAs (A), and PCAs (P) are seen in the same plane in this example.

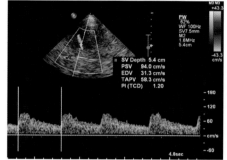

Mean velocity (TAPV in this scanner) and pulsatility index in a healthy adult MCA.

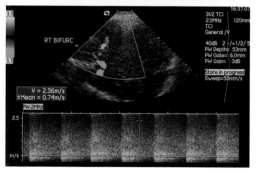

Middle cerebral artery velocities in a child with sickle cell disease. Velocities are high and the sonogram weak; a single cursor has been placed to estimate the mean of the maximum velocity envelope. Note that no angle correction is used. A mean velocity of 236 cm/s is indicative of stenosis.

MEASUREMENTS

The main measurements for TCD applications are TCD mean velocity and Pulsatility Index (PI).

$$PI = \frac{\text{Peak Systolic Velocity} - \text{End Diastolic Velocity}}{\text{Time Averaged Maximum Velocity}}$$

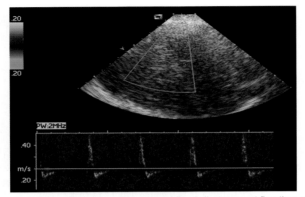

A sharp spike in MCA velocity followed by reversed flow indicates no net flow through the artery consistent with brain death.

TCD mean velocity is measured from the outline of the spectral display over one or more cardiac cycles and is described as Time Averaged Maximum, Time Averaged Maximum Mean, or Time Averaged Peak, depending on the scanner (see image on page 173).

Transcranial Doppler studies are conducted with both non-imaging TCD and imaging TCD (TCDi). Much of the literature and data for TCD applications are based on non-imaging TCD where angle correction is not possible. Operators using duplex scanners should not make beam/vessel angle corrections and should optimize the Doppler trace by moving the probe to align the vessel with the Doppler beam as best as possible.

Mean and standard deviation (SD) adult normal intracranial mean velocities (cm/s)

	< 40 years (± SD)	40–59 years (± SD)	> 60 years (± SD)
MCA (M1)	58.4 ± 8.4	57.7 ± 11.5	44.7 ± 11.1
ACA (A1)	47.3 ± 13.6	53.1 ± 10.5	45.3 ± 13.5
PCA (P1)	34.2 ± 7.8	36.6 ± 9.8	29.9 ± 9.3
VA/BA	34.9 ± 7.8	36.4 ± 11.7	30.5 ± 12.4

MCA, middle cerebral artery; ACA, anterior cerebral artery; PCA, posterior cerebral artery; VA, vertebral artery; BA, basilar artery.

Mean and standard deviation (SD) adult normal intracranial pulsatility indices (PI)

Arteries	Pulsatility index (± SD)
R MCA	0.90 ± 0.24
L MCA	0.94 ± 0.27
R ACA	0.78 ± 0.15
L ACA	0.83 ± 0.17
R PCA	0.88 ± 0.23
L PCA	0.88 ± 0.20

Mean and standard deviation (SD) children normal intracranial mean velocities (cm/s)

	1.0–2.9 years	3.0–5.9 years	6.0–9.9 years	10–18 years
MCA (M1)	85 ± 10	94 ± 10	97 ± 9	81 ± 11
ACA (A1)	55 ± 13	71 ± 5	65 ± 13	56 ± 14
PCA (P1)	50 ± 17	56 ± 13	57 ± 9	50 ± 10
VA/BA	51 ± 6	58 ± 6	58 ± 9	46 ± 8

Applications

There is a wide range of applications for TCD, and readers are advised to consult specialist texts before embarking on studies or clinical practice.

Applications include:
• Screening for stroke risk in children with sickle disease
• Detection and monitoring of angiographic vasospasm after spontaneous subarachnoid hemorrhage
• Evaluation of intracranial stenosis (MCA and distal ICA)
• Confirmatory test, in support of a clinical diagnosis of brain death
• Microembolism detection
• Vasomotor reactivity testing
• Detection of raised intracranial pressure.

Evidence for the efficacy of each has been summarized by the American Academy of Neurology. Applications for which there is strong evidence of clinical effectiveness include the following.

Screening for stroke risk in children with sickle cell disease
Children should be screened annually from 18–24 months to 16 years. Distal ICA, MCA, ACA, and PCA velocities are measured.

	Velocities (cm/s)	Category
dICA, MCA, ACA, PCA	< 170	Normal
dICA, MCA, ACA*	170–199	Conditional
dICA, MCA	≥ 200	Abnormal

*ACA velocities of ≥ 170 cm/s have also been described as indicating abnormal hemodynamics and are associated with increased risk of stroke.

MCA velocities of < 70 cm/s with MCA (lower/higher side) ratio of ≤ 0.5 are indicative of anomalies, as is the absence of MCA signals in the presence of a good ultrasound window.

Children in the normal category are usually monitored annually, and those in the conditional category are scanned at an earlier date depending on values and clinical judgement. Children with abnormal velocities should have early (within 2 weeks) repeat scans with additional imaging (MRI/A) with a view to treatment.

Detection and monitoring of angiographic vasospasm after spontaneous subarachnoid hemorrhage (SAH)
Daily measurement of MCA velocity is made in patients with risk of vasospasm following SAH. Proximal vasospasm leads to increases in mean velocity. Distal vasospasm leads to an increase in resistance evident in increased pulsatility. There is variation between patients, but unfavorable signs include:
- Early appearance of MCA mean velocity ≥ 180 cm/s
- Rapid (> 20% or > 65 cm/s) daily increase in mean velocity from days 3–7
- MCA/ICA ratio ≥ 6
- Abrupt appearance of high pulsatility (PI > 1.5).

Detection of brain death

TCD can rule out cerebral circulatory arrest if positive diastolic flow is detected. It can confirm brain death by demonstrating complete cerebral circulatory arrest in anterior and posterior circulations.

FURTHER READING

Adams RJ, McKie VC, Hsu L, Files B, Vichinsky E, Pegelow C, Abboud M, Gallagher D, Kutlar A, Nichols FT, Bonds DR, Brambilla D. Prevention of a first stroke by transfusions in children with sickle cell anemia and abnormal results on transcranial Doppler ultrasonography. *New Engl J Med.* 1998; 339:5–11.

Alexandrov AV, Sloan MA, Tegeler CH, Newell DN, Lumsden A, Garami Z, Levy CR, Wong LKS, Douville C, Kaps M, Tsivgoulis G, Practice standards for transcranial Doppler (TCD) ultrasound—Part II. Clinical indications and expected outcomes. *J Neuroimaging.* 2012; 22:215–224.

Bode H, Wais U. Age dependence on flow velocities in basal cerebral arteries. *Arch Dis Child.* 1988; 63:606–611.

Hennerici M, Rautenberg W, Sitzer G, Schwarz A. Transcranial Doppler ultrasound for the assessment of intracranial arterial flow velocity—Part 1 examination technique and normal values. *Surg Neurol.* 1987; 27:439–448

Kwiatowski JL, Granger S, Brambilla DJ, Brown RC, Miller ST, Adams RJ. Elevated blood flow velocity in the anterior cerebral artery and stroke risk in sickle cell disease: Extended analysis from the STOP trial. *Br J Haematology.* 2006; 134:333–339.

Sloan MA, Alexandrov AV, Tegeler CH, Spencer MP, Caplan LR, Feldmann E, Wechsler LR, Newell DW, Gomez CR, Babikian VL, Lefkowitz D, Goldman RS, Armon C, Hsu CY, Goodin DS. Therapeutics and Technology Assessment Subcommittee of the American Academy of Neurology. Assessment: Transcranial Doppler ultrasonography: report of the Therapeutics and Technology Assessment Subcommittee of the American Academy of Neurology. *Neurology.* 2004; 62:1468–1481.

8 PERIPHERAL VASCULAR (VENOUS)

*Colin R. Deane and
Paul S. Sidhu*

Inferior vena cava (IVC)

PREPARATION
None.

POSITION
Supine.

PROBE
1.0–5.0 MHz curvilinear transducer.

METHOD
The patient is examined in three phases:
1. Quiet respiration
2. During breath holding (Valsalva maneuver)
3. On leg raising

Examine in the transverse plane in the epigastrium and measure the short and long axis diameter 1 cm below the level of the left renal vein.

APPEARANCES
A tubular structure lying to the right of the midline with variable diameter with respiratory cycle.

MEASUREMENTS

Mean IVC diameter	
Phase	**Diameter in mm (range)**
During quiet respiration	17.2 (5.1–28.9)
During breath holding	18.8 (7.7–31.3)
During leg raising	17.6 (9.7–31.0)

Measurement of the proximal IVC has been proposed as a measure of patient intravascular volume status. Diameter and change in IVC diameter is measured 2–3 cm before the confluence with the right atrium. B-mode and M-mode measurements are used. There are pitfalls in the test, and it should be used with caution in clinical practice for this critical application.

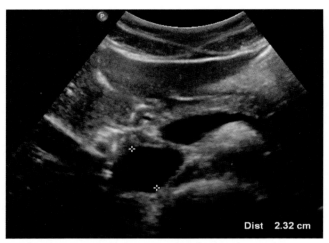

Vena cava diameter—an approximate measurement of an irregular vessel.

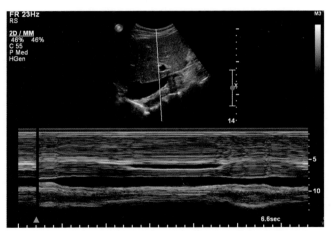

The proximal vena cava. M-mode shows changes in diameter with inspiration and expiration. Care must be taken to ensure that translational movement does not cause over- or underestimation of change in diameter.

FURTHER READING

Sykes AM, McLoughlin RF, So CBB, Cooperberg PL, Mathieson JR, Gray RR, Brandt R. Sonographic assessment of infrarenal inferior vena caval dimensions. *J Ultrasound Med*. 1995; 4:665–668.

Neck veins

PREPARATION
None.

POSITION
Supine.

PROBE
5.0–8.0 MHz linear transducer.

METHOD
Both longitudinal and transverse planes to examine the vessels. Spectral Doppler measurements are made in the longitudinal plane with angle correction applied.

APPEARANCES
The vessel lumen is echo-free, the veins are compressible, and the venous confluence is Y-shaped. The diameter is dependent on head position relative to the heart. Blood flow is symmetrical and biphasic in 57%, continuous and monophasic in 29%, and monophasic in 13%. Velocity is less than 100 cm/sec at mid-neck and is variable depending on the head position and pressure of the transducer. Velocities become markedly more pulsatile in the proximal internal jugular vein (IJV).

MEASUREMENTS

Flow velocities in neck veins

Measurement location	Velocity (cm/sec ± SD) Mean ± SD
Right internal jugular	28 ± 15
Right innominate	33 ± 16
Right subclavian	16 ± 10
Left internal jugular	22 ± 16
Left innominate	22 ± 11
Left subclavian	11 ± 7

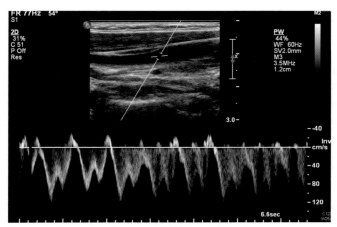

The proximal jugular vein shows velocity changes as a result of pressure changes in the right atrium.

FURTHER READING

Clenaghan S, McLaughlin RE, Martyn C, McGovern S, Bowra J. Relationship between Trendelenburg tilt and internal jugular vein diameter. *Emerg Med J*. 2005; 22:867–868.

Pucheu A, Evans J, Thomas D, Scheuble C, Pucheu M. Doppler ultrasonography of normal neck veins. *J Clin Ultrasound*. 1994; 22:367–373.

Leg veins

PREPARATION
None.

POSITION
Supine.

PROBE
3.0–8.0 MHz linear array transducer. 1.0–5.0 MHz curvilinear arrays may be useful in large patients.

METHOD
Measurements are performed at the common femoral vein, high superficial femoral vein, midsuperficial femoral vein, low superficial femoral vein, and the popliteal vein. Anteroposterior measurements are taken in the transverse plane. A vein-to-artery ratio can be calculated from an arterial measurement at the same level as the vein measurement. Veins with an acute thrombosis are larger and veins with a chronic thrombosis are smaller than normal veins. There is considerable overlap in the measurements.

For scans for deep vein thrombosis, exclusion of thrombus at the site of measurement is confirmed by complete compression of the vein in a transverse view. Note that the term superficial femoral vein is not used to report for the presence or absence of DVT. Femoral vein is preferred to avoid confusion.

APPEARANCES
The veins of the legs are identified as echo-poor structures that are readily compressible with a continuous forward spectral Doppler trace with some respiratory or right atrial pressure modulation.

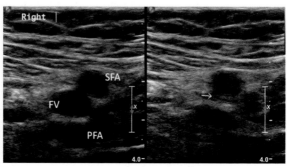

Compression of the femoral vein (right) shows complete collapse (arrow), while the arteries remain relatively unaffected. This demonstrates absence of thrombus at the measurement site.

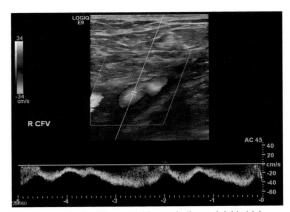

Normal femoral vein velocity changes caused by respiration and right atrial pressure changes.

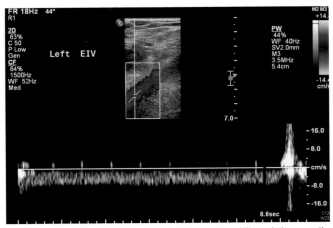

Absence of respiration changes in a common femoral or external iliac vein is suggestive of proximal obstruction, in this case a common iliac vein thrombus.

MEASUREMENTS

Vein-to-artery ratio is calculated by dividing the anteroposterior vein diameter by the anteroposterior artery diameter at the same point.

Vessel	Vein diameter Mean ± SD (mm)	Vein/artery ratio Mean ± SD
Common femoral vein	10.57 ± 2.88	1.34 ± 0.37
High superficial femoral vein	7.10 ± 1.96	1.24 ± 0.36
Mid superficial femoral vein	6.41 ± 1.72	1.21 ± 0.33
Low superficial femoral vein	6.52 ± 1.74	1.19 ± 0.32
Popliteal femoral vein	6.80 ± 2.11	1.22 ± 0.36

(From Hertzberg BS et al., 1997)

Diameter increases with increased reverse Trendelenburg tilt and increases by 20% during a Valsalva maneuver.

Velocities are variable depending on patient position and flow to the lower limb. Common femoral and external iliac venous waveforms show respiratory or right heart variations. Absence of velocity variation, especially in the presence of variation in the contralateral limb, is indicative of proximal venous obstruction.

FURTHER READING

Fronek A, Criqui MH, Denenberg J, Langer RD. Common femoral vein dimensions and hemodynamics including Valsalva response as a function of sex, age, and ethnicity in a population study. *J Vasc Surg.* 2001; 33:1050–1056.

Hertzberg BS, Kliewer MA, DeLong DM, Lalouche KJ, Paulson EK, Frederick MG, Carroll BA. Sonographic assessment of lower limb vein diameters: Implications for the diagnosis and characterization of deep venous thrombosis. *AJR Am J Roentgenol.* 1997; 168:1253–1257.

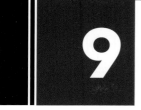

9

MUSCULOSKELETAL SYSTEM

Bhavna Batohi,
Keshthra Satchithananda, and
David Elias

GENERAL CONSIDERATIONS

PREPARATION
None.

POSITION
See individual examinations.

TRANSDUCER
- High-resolution, high-quality ultrasound equipment.
- >10 MHz linear transducer for small superficial structures; ideally, a hockey stick transducer.
- 7.0–18.0 MHz linear transducers for tendons of extremities.
- 3.5–8.0 MHz linear transducers to image large or deep muscles.

Linear probes ideal to provide uniform field of view with superior near-field resolution.

METHOD
See individual examinations.

APPEARANCES
1. Muscles are of low reflectivity with high-reflective intramuscular fibro-adipose septae, perimuscular epimysium, and intermuscular fascia.
2. Tendons consist of parallel fascicles of collagen fibers, which appear as parallel high-reflective lines due to multiple reflective interfaces. Most tendons are lined by a synovial sheath, which contains a thin film of fluid. This appears as a low-reflective rim normally < 2 mm thick. Those without a sheath (e.g., tendon Achilles) have a surrounding high-reflective line due to the dense connective tissue of the epitendineum.
3. Ligaments have more interweaved and irregular collagen fibers than tendons and thus appear as 2–3 mm thick homogeneous high-reflective bands.
4. Normal bursae appear as a low-reflective line, representing fluid, surrounded by a high-reflective line.
5. Peripheral nerves exhibit parallel linear internal echoes on longitudinal images. On transverse images, nerves are round or oval structures with tiny punctate internal echoes.

MEASUREMENTS

Comparisons should be made with the joint or structure on the opposite limb. For specific measurements, see individual examinations.

ARTIFACTS

Anisotropy occurs in tissues composed of parallel linear fibers. It is an artifact created by an apparent reduction in echogenicity when the angle of insonation deviates from being perpendicular to the plane of the linear fibers. Tendons are markedly anisotropic; nerves, muscles, and ligaments moderately so. For all these tissues, the angle of insonation should remain close to perpendicular to the fibers to demonstrate a normal reflective ultrasound appearance. Loss of perpendicularity results in artifactually low reflectivity. For superficial tendons with a curved overlying skin surface, the use of a stand-off pad, or imaging of structures in a water bath (e.g., for finger tendons), can be helpful to allow maintenance of probe contact with the skin and at the same time keep a perpendicular insonation angle. Alternatively, modern units, which allow beam steering or compound imaging, may be helpful in reducing anisotropic artifact.

FURTHER READING

Bianchi S, et al. *Ultrasound of the Musculoskeletal System.* Berlin: Springer-Verlag Berlin and Heidelberg GmbH & Co. K, 2004.

McNally E. *Practical Musculoskeletal Ultrasound.* London: Churchill Livingstone, 2014.

O'Neill J. *Musculoskeletal Ultrasound Anatomy and Technique.* New York: Springer, 2008.

UPPER LIMB: SHOULDER

Long head of biceps

PREPARATION
None.

POSITION
The patient is imaged while seated. The humerus is in a neutral position with the elbow flexed and hand, with palm up, resting on patient's lap.

TRANSDUCER
7.0–10.0 MHz linear transducer.

METHOD
The transducer is placed transversely and longitudinally across bicipital groove on the anterior aspect of the shoulder.

APPEARANCES
- Transverse section: The long head of the biceps (LHB) tendon is a high-reflective ovoid structure within bicipital groove. This is an important view to detect intra-articular fluid around the LHB tendon. Measurements are made in the transverse plane of the width of the long head of the biceps within the bicipital groove.
- Longitudinal section: Should identify the fibrillary echo pattern of the tendon.

MEASUREMENTS

	Dominant (mean ± SD)	Nondominant (mean ± SD)
Male	3.4 ± 0.4 mm	3.3 ± 0.6 mm
Female	2.9 ± 0.4 mm	2.9 ± 0.4 mm

FURTHER READING
Allen, GM. Shoulder ultrasound imaging—integrating anatomy, biomechanics and disease processes. *Eur J Radiol*. 2008; 68: 137–146.
Beggs S. Shoulder Ultrasound. *Semin Ultrasound CT MRI*. 2011; 32:101–113.

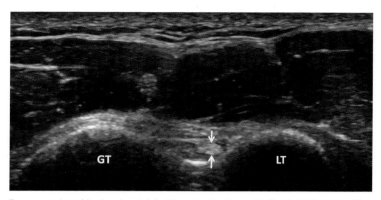

Transverse view of the long head of the biceps tendon (arrows) in the bicipital groove of the humerus (GT, greater tuberosity; LT, lesser tuberosity).

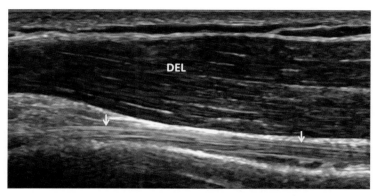

Longitudinal view of the long head of the biceps tendon (arrows). (DEL, deltoid)

Karthikeyan S, Rai SB, Parsons H, Drew S, Smith CD, Griffin DR. Ultrasound dimensions of the rotator cuff in young healthy adults. *J Shoulder Elbow Surg.* 2014; 23: 1107–1112.

Subscapularis tendon

PREPARATION
None.

POSITION
The patient is imaged while seated. The humerus is externally rotated to stretch the subscapularis tendon. The probe is placed lateral to the coracoid.

TRANSDUCER
7.0–10.0 MHz linear transducer.

METHOD
The transducer is placed transversely and longitudinally across the subscapularis tendon, which lies medial to the bicipital groove inserting into the lesser tuberosity.

APPEARANCES
The subscapularis tendon has a convex margin superficially and follows the convex humeral cortex on its deep aspect. Transverse to the tendon, the multipenate anatomy of the tendon may be appreciated. Small subdeltoid effusions may be apparent superficial to subscapularis.

FURTHER READING
Middleton WD, Teefey SA, Yamaguchi K. Sonography of the shoulder. *Sem Musculoskeletal Radiol.* 1998; 211:211–222.

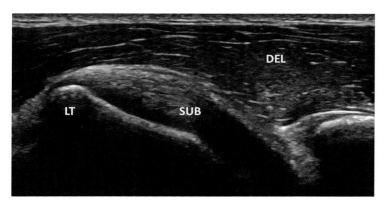

Longitudinal view of the subscapularis tendon (SUB) as it attaches to the lesser tuberosity (LT).

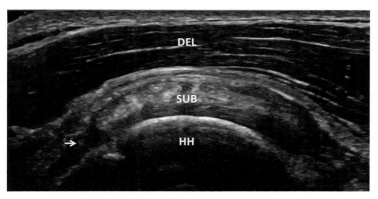

Transverse view of the subscapularis tendon (SUB) showing its multipenate structure adjacent to the long head of the biceps (arrow). (DEL, deltoid; HH, humeral head)

Supraspinatus tendon

PREPARATION
None.

POSITION
The patient is imaged while seated. The humerus is extended and internally rotated with the hand on the ipsilateral hip and then the "hand in opposite back pocket" position.

TRANSDUCER
7.0–10.0 MHz linear transducer.

METHOD
The transducer placed transversely and longitudinally across the supraspinatus tendon.

APPEARANCES
- Transverse section: High reflectivity fibrillary pattern of tendon fibers with a smoothly convex superficial contour deep to the deltoid and subdeltoid fat stripe. The tendon lies superficial to the low-reflective cartilage of the humeral head.
- Longitudinal section: The tendon is thick as it emerges from under the acromion and thins distally as it inserts into the greater tuberosity. This results in a triangular shape.

MEASUREMENTS

	Maximum anteroposterior width at foot plate (mean ± SD)	Thickness from bursal surface to articular cartilage (mean ± SD)
Male	14.9 ± 1.5 mm	5.8 ± 0.9 mm
Female	13.5 ± 1.2 mm	5.0 ± 0.6 mm

FURTHER READING
Karthikeyan S, Rai SB, Parsons H, Drew S, Smith CD, Griffin DR. Ultrasound dimensions of the rotator cuff in young healthy adults. *J Shoulder Elbow Surg.* 2014; 23:1107–1112.

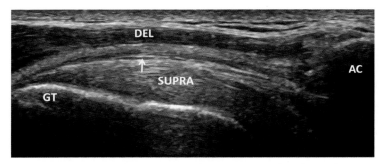

Longitudinal view of the supraspinatus tendon (SUPRA) as emerges from deep to the acromion and inserts onto the greater tuberosity. The hypoechoic line above the tendon is the subdeltoid bursa (arrow). (AC, acromion; DEL, deltoid; GT, greater tuberosity)

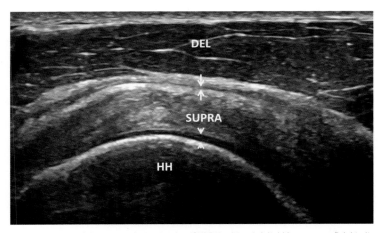

Transverse view of the supraspinatus tendon (SUPRA) with subdeltoid bursa superficial to it (arrows). Articular cartilage of the humeral head is hypoechoic (arrowheads).

Infraspinatus tendon

PREPARATION
None.

POSITION
The patient is imaged while seated. The ipsilateral hand is placed on the contralateral shoulder to stretch out the infraspinatus. The transducer is placed on the posterior shoulder, inferior and parallel to the scapular spine, sweeping laterally to identify the muscle belly and then tendon.

TRANSDUCER
7.0–10.0 MHz linear transducer.

METHOD
The transducer is placed transversely and longitudinally across the infraspinatus.

APPEARANCES
The infraspinatus tendon appears as an elongated soft tissue triangle that attaches to greater tuberosity of the humerus. The infraspinatus tendon needs to be differentiated from teres minor tendon. The latter is inferior to the infraspinatus tendon and appears trapezoidal with fibers that run obliquely as opposed to horizontal lines of infraspinatus tendon.

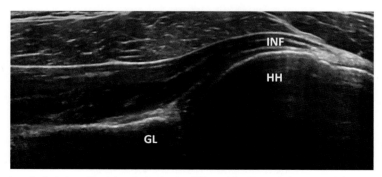

Longitudinal view of the infraspinatus tendon (INF) overlying the posterior aspect of the humeral head (HH) and glenoid (GL).

FURTHER READING

Karthikeyan S, Rai SB, Parsons H, Drew S, Smith CD, Griffin DR. Ultrasound dimensions of the rotator cuff in young healthy adults. *J Shoulder Elbow Surg.* 2014; 23:1107–1112.

UPPER LIMB: ELBOW

Anterior joint space and distal biceps tendon

PREPARATION
None.

POSITION
The patient is seated with the forearm supinated and elbow initially slightly flexed.

TRANSDUCER
10.0–15.0 MHz linear transducer.

METHOD
The anterior joint space is imaged in longitudinal section with the elbow fully extended and the transducer over the anterior radiocapitellar joint. The distal biceps tendon is imaged in longitudinal and transverse section with the elbow slightly flexed. It is often difficult to fully visualize due to anisotropy in this position. The elbow is then flexed to 70°–80° and the distal biceps tendon is identified through a window from the anteromedial elbow. The very distal biceps tendon is imaged by completely flexing the elbow and pronating the forearm in a "cobra position" and scanning in transverse section along the dorsal proximal forearm.

APPEARANCE
The anterior capsule of the elbow joint is a high-reflective line that follows the ventral contours of the proximal radial head and distal humeral capitellum. Between the capsule and the bone lies a 1-mm-thick, low-reflective layer representing articular cartilage, which should not be mistaken for abnormal joint fluid. The distal biceps tendon appears as a highly reflective fibrillary structure extending from the musculotendinous junction of the biceps to the radial tuberosity.

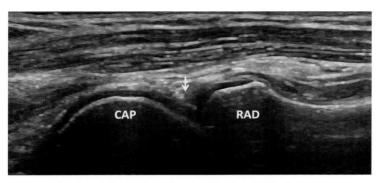

Transverse view through the anterior joint space of the elbow (RAD, radius; CAP, capitellum). The arrow points to the anterior synovial recess, where the joint may be evaluated for the presence of an effusion.

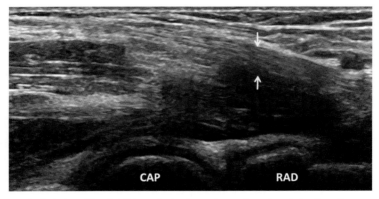

Longitudinal view of the distal biceps tendon (arrows) seen through a window from the anteromedial elbow (RAD, radius; CAP, capitellum).

MEASUREMENTS
Please note that these are cadaveric measurements.

Mean width distal biceps tendon (range)	Mean length distal biceps tendon (range)
7 mm (6–10 mm)	21 mm (17–25 mm)

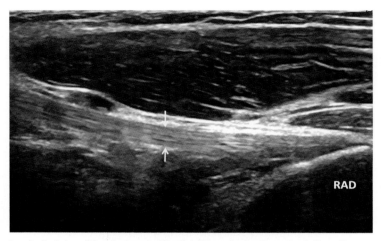

Longitudinal view of the attachment of the distal biceps tendon (arrows) onto the radius (RAD).

FURTHER READING

Athwal GS, Steinmann SP and Rispoli. The distal biceps tendon: Footprint and relevant clinical anatomy. *J Hand Surg.* 2007; 32A:1225–1229.

Brasseur JL. The biceps tendons: From the top and from the bottom. *J Ultrasound.* 2012; 15:29–38.

De Maeseneer M, Marcelis S, Cattrysse E, Shahabpour M, De Smet K, De Mey J. Ultrasound of the elbow: A systematic approach using bony landmarks. *Eur J Radiol.* 2012; 81:919–922.

Olecranon fossa, ulnar nerve, and distal triceps

PREPARATION
None.

POSITION
For the olecranon fossa and distal triceps, the patient is seated with the elbow flexed at 90° in a "crab" position with the palm resting on the table. The ulnar nerve can be visualized in the crab position or with the elbow extended and the arm outstretched.

TRANSDUCER
10.0–15.0 MHz linear transducer.

METHOD
The distal triceps tendon is imaged in longitudinal and transverse section. Deep to the distal triceps, the olecranon fossa and posterior fat pad can be seen in longitudinal and transverse section. The ulnar nerve is visualized in transverse section within the cubital tunnel, just dorsal to the medial epicondyle. Once identified, the nerve can be visualized in longitudinal section also.

APPEARANCE
Within the olecranon fossa is the posterior fat pad. The cubital tunnel and ulnar nerve can also be identified. The ulnar nerve is fascicular in appearance but in the cubital tunnel is hypoechoic.

MEASUREMENTS
Mean cross-sectional area of the ulnar nerve at the cubital tunnel 0.065 ± 0.01 cm^2.

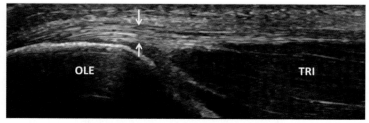

Longitudinal view of the triceps muscle (TRI) and distal triceps tendon (arrows) as it inserts onto the olecranon (OLE).

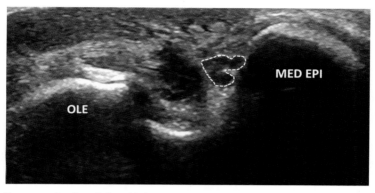

Transverse view through the cubital tunnel bordered by the medial epicondyle (MED EPI) and (olecranon). The ulna nerve (dashed line) is positioned adjacent to the medial epicondyle and its cross-sectional area can be assessed in this position.

FURTHER READING

Wiesler ER, Chloros GD, Cartwright MS, Shin HW, Walker FO. Ultrasound in the diagnosis of ulnar neuropathy at the cubital tunnel. *J Hand Surg Am.* 2006; 31:1088–1093.

Lateral elbow

PREPARATION
None.

POSITION
Patient seated with elbows flexed and resting on the table.

TRANSDUCER
10.0–15.0 MHz linear transducer.

METHOD
The transducer is placed over the lateral epicondyle in the plane of the common extensor tendon origin.

APPEARANCE
The common extensor tendon arises from the lateral epicondyle of the humerus. The radial collateral ligament lies deep to the tendon and attaches to the annular ligament at the radial head. The lateral ulnar collateral ligament forms a sling around the posterior radial neck to insert into the proximal ulna. These ligaments may be followed from their origin at the lateral epicondyle. The radiocapitellar joint is seen and can be assessed for the presence of fluid.

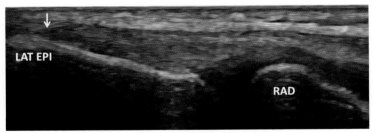

The common forearm extensor origin (arrow) arises from the lateral epicondyle of the humerus (LAT EPI) and lies superior to the radial head (RAD).

FURTHER READING
Radunovic G, Vlad V, Micu MC, Nestorova R, Petranova T, Porta F, Iagnocco A. Ultrasound assessment of the elbow. *Med Ultrason.* 2012; 14:141–146.

Medial elbow

PREPARATION
None.

POSITION
Patient seated with elbows extended on a table.

TRANSDUCER
10.0–15.0 MHz linear transducer.

METHOD
The transducer is placed in the longitudinal oblique position at the medial elbow joint.

APPEARANCE
The common flexor tendon arises at the medial epicondyle of the humerus. The anterior band of the ulnar collateral ligament arises from the medial epicondyle of the humerus and inserts on the medial coronoid process of the ulna.

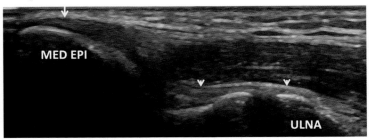

The common flexor tendon origin (arrow) arises from the medial epicondyle (MED EPI) of the humerus. Anterior band of the ulna collateral ligament (arrowheads).

FURTHER READING
Radunovic G, Vlad V, Micu MC, Nestorova R, Petranova T, Porta F, Iagnocco A. Ultrasound assessment of the elbow. *Med Ultrason.* 2012; 14:141–146.

UPPER LIMB: WRIST

Dorsal tendons

PREPARATION
None.

POSITION
Palm placed face down on examination table.

TRANSDUCER
10.0–15.0 MHz linear transducer.

METHOD
The transducer is placed transversely across the wrist at the level of the dorsal radial tubercle, Lister's tubercle, and then moved to follow individual tendons. Each tendon is then examined transversely and longitudinally.

APPEARANCE
The dorsal tendons course through six separate synovial compartments. The dorsal radial tubercle acts as an anatomical landmark separating the extensor pollicis longus, which lies on its ulnar side, from the extensor carpi radialis brevis and longus, which lie on its radial side.

MEASUREMENTS

Compartments

Radial side

1. Abductor pollicis longus tendon (forms the volar margin of anatomical snuff box) and extensor pollicus brevis tendon (lies deep in the anatomical snuff box)
2. Extensor carpi radialis longus and extensor carpi radialis brevis tendons
3. Extensor pollicus longus tendon (forms dorsal margin of anatomical snuff box and crosses over ECRL/ ECRB radially, distal to Lister's tubercle)
4. Extensor digitorum and extensor indicis tendons
5. Extensor digiti minimi tendon

Ulnar side

6. Extensor carpi ulnaris tendon lying in a groove on the medial ulna

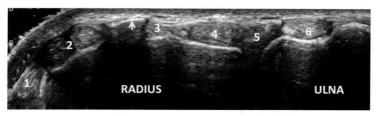

Transverse view of the dorsal tendons of the wrist. 1, APL and EPB; 2, ECRL and ECRB; 3, EPL on the ulnar aspect of Lister's tubercle (arrow); 4, ED and EI; 5, EDM; 6, ECU lying in a groove on distal ulna.

FURTHER READING

Klauser AS, Halpern EJ, De Zordo T, Feuchtner GM, Arora R, Gruber J, Martinoli C, Löscher WN. Carpal tunnel syndrome assessment with US: Value of additional cross-sectional area measurements of the median nerve in patients versus healthy volunteers. *Radiology.* 2009; 250: 171–177.

Min-Kyu Kim MK, Jeon HJ, Park SH, Park DS, Nam HS. Value of ultrasonography in the diagnosis of carpal tunnel syndrome: Correlation with electrophysiological abnormalities and clinical severity. *J Korean Neurosurg Soc.* 2014; 55:78–82.

Sofka CM. Ultrasound of the hand and wrist. *Ultrasound Quarterly.* 2014; 30: 184–192.

Carpal tunnel

PREPARATION
None.

POSITION
Patient seated with palm face up on the examination table.

TRANSDUCER
10.0–15.0 MHz linear transducer.

METHOD
The transducer is placed transversely and then longitudinally across the volar wrist at the level of the distal carpal crease.

APPEARANCE
The floor of the carpal tunnel is formed by the carpal bones and its roof by the flexor retinaculum, which attaches to the scaphoid tubercle and the trapezium laterally and the pisiform and hook of hamate medially. The median nerve lies just deep to the retinaculum at the radial aspect of the carpal tunnel. Also within the tunnel lie the flexor digitorum superficialis and profundus tendons, and within its radial aspect, flexor pollicis longus and flexor carpi radialis. Superficial to the ulna side of the carpal tunnel lies Guyon's canal containing the ulna nerve and artery. Flexor carpi ulnaris lies medially and inserts into the pisiform. Identification of the median nerve is aided by noting that in the distal forearm it lies deep to flexor digitorum superficialis, and more distally it courses around the radial aspect of these tendons to reach the superficial carpal tunnel. In addition, it shows less movement on finger flexion/extension than the flexor tendons. The cross-sectional area of the nerve should be measured at the distal carpal crease (i.e., the level of the pisiform and scaphoid tubercle). The wrist should be in neutral position for a reproducible measurement.

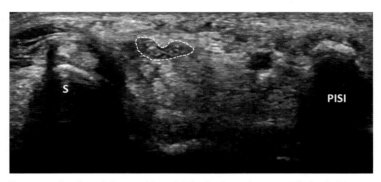

Transverse view through the carpal tunnel at the distal carpal crease, at the level of the pisiform (PISI), showing the median nerve in cross-section (dashed line). (S, distal scaphoid)

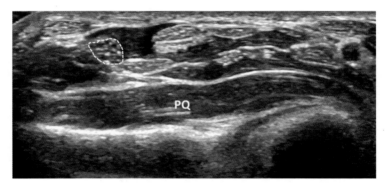

Transverse view of the median nerve (dashed line) at the level of the pronator quadratus (PQ).

MEASUREMENTS

Improved diagnostic accuracy is obtained by determining the difference in the cross-sectional area of the median nerve at the carpal tunnel and level of pronator quadratus.

Normal mean cross-sectional area at the distal carpal crease ($\pm$ SD)	Difference between cross-sectional area at the distal carpal crease and level of pronator quadratus
9.0 mm^2 ($\pm$ 1.5 mm^2)	0.25 mm^2 ($\pm$0.43 mm^2)

FURTHER READING

Klauser AS, Halpern EJ, De Zordo T, Feuchtner GM, Arora R, Gruber J, Martinoli C, Löscher WN. Carpal tunnel syndrome assessment with US: Value of additional cross-sectional area measurements of the median nerve in patients versus healthy volunteers. *Radiology.* 2009; 250:171–177.

Min-Kyu Kim MK, Jeon HJ, Park SH, Park DS, Nam HS. Value of ultrasonography in the diagnosis of carpal tunnel syndrome: Correlation with electrophysiological abnormalities and clinical severity. *J Korean Neurosurg Soc.* 2014; 55:78–82.

Sofka CM. Ultrasound of the hand and wrist. *Ultrasound Quarterly.* 2014; 30:184–192.

LOWER LIMB: HIPS

Hip effusion

PREPARATION
None.

POSITION
Supine.

TRANSDUCER
7.0–10.0 MHz linear transducer dependent on patient's age.

METHOD
The transducer is placed along the length of the femoral neck.

APPEARANCE
The high-reflective anterior capsule is identified anterior to the femoral neck.

MEASUREMENTS
In children, separation of the capsule from the femoral neck is normally 2–4 mm, and a difference of 2 mm or more between symptomatic and asymptomatic sides is considered significant for a joint effusion.

In adults, the distance of the capsule from the femoral neck is normally < 7 mm, and a difference of 1 mm or more between symptomatic and asymptomatic sides is considered significant for a joint effusion.

FURTHER READING

Bierma-Zeinstra SM, Bohnen AM, Verhaar JA, Prins A, Ginai-Karamat AZ, Laméris JS. Sonography for hip joint effusion in adults with hip pain. *Ann Rheum Dis*. 2000; 59:178–182.

Rohrschnieder WK, Fuchs G, Troger J. Ultrasonographic evaluation of the anterior recess in the normal hip: A prospective study on 166 asymptomatic children. *Pediat Radiol*. 1006; 26: 629–634.

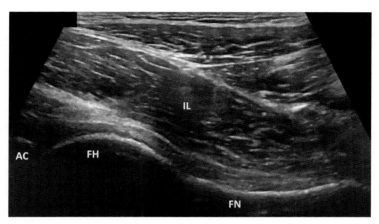

Hip joint effusion can be assessed by measuring the distance between the femoral neck (FN) and anterior joint capsule (not seen on this normal hip). (AC, acetabulum; FH, femoral head; IL, iliopsoas muscle).

Developmental dysplasia of the hip

PREPARATION
None.

POSITION
The patient is placed in a right and left lateral decubitus position for examination of each hip; ideally in a cradle.

TRANSDUCER
Linear transducer; 7.5 MHz (newborn), 5.0–7.5 MHz (3 months).

METHOD
The infant should be as relaxed as possible (recent feed, parental presence, and examination in a darkened room are helpful). Each position is assessed in the coronal plane by placing the transducer longitudinally at the lateral hip. A static examination is performed with the hip in a neutral position. For dynamic examination the hip is flexed at 90° and gently adducted and abducted, and gentle posteriorly directed stress is applied to the flexed, adducted hip.

APPEARANCE
On coronal images the iliac wing is seen as a horizontal high-reflective line paralleling the transducer. The bony acetabulum forms a high-reflective curve medially with a defect representing the normal triradiate cartilage. Prior to ossification the femoral head is low reflective with scattered specular echoes due to vascular channels. Superolateral to the femoral head the joint capsule is seen as a high-reflective line attaching to the ilium. Just deep to this a small high-reflective focus represents condensed fibrocartilage at the labral tip. The remaining labrum is seen as low-reflective cartilage similar in reflectivity to the femoral head.

MEASUREMENTS
1. Graf alpha angle: Angle between the iliac line and a line along the osseous acetabular roof on a coronal image of the hip. Normal is > 60°.
2. Femoral head coverage: Relative coverage of the femoral head by the bony acetabulum in flexion. Normal is > 58%.

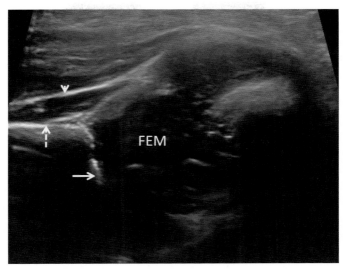

Coronal view through the pediatric hip showing the low-reflective femoral head (FEM) with scattered specular echoes lying appropriately in the acetabulum. (Dashed arrow, Iliac wing; solid arrow, bony acetabulum; arrow head, joint capsule)

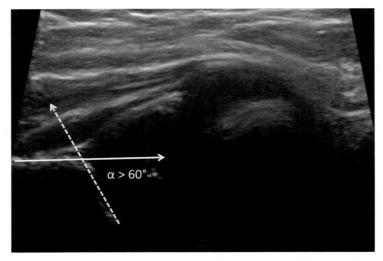

Coronal view through the pediatric hip showing the Graf alpha angle, which is measured between the iliac line (solid arrow) and osseous acetabular roof (dashed arrow).

FURTHER READING

Graf R. Fundamentals of sonographic diagnosis of infant hip dysplasia. *J Pediatr Ortho*. 1984; 4:735–740.

Morin C, Harcke HT, MacEwen GD. The infant hip: Real-time US assessment of acetabular development. *Radiology*. 1985; 157:673–677.

Ömeroğlu, H. Use of ultrasonography in developmental dysplasia of the hip. *J Child Orthop*. 2014; 8:105–113.

LOWER LIMB: KNEE

Anterior knee

PREPARATION
None.

POSITION
Supine for anterior structures with the knee extended for assessment of collateral ligaments. Quadriceps and patellar tendons are examined in flexion and extension. Measurement of fluid in the suprapatellar pouch should be performed with the knee flexed at 30°.

TRANSDUCER
7.0–15.0 MHz linear transducer.

METHOD
The presence of joint fluid should be sought in the suprapatellar bursa and the medial and lateral joint recesses. The quadriceps and patellar tendons, and medial and lateral collateral ligaments are evaluated in transversal and longitudinal planes.

APPEARANCE
The suprapatellar pouch is a low-reflective band above the patella and deep to the quadriceps tendon. It lies between the suprapatellar and pre-femoral fat pads.

The medial collateral ligament has superficial and deep components. The superficial ligament attaches to the medial epicondyle of the femur and the medial tibial metaphysis.

The lateral ligamentous structures include the iliotibial band anteriorly, which inserts onto the anterolateral tibia; the fibular collateral ligament, which runs obliquely from the lateral epicondyle of the femur to insert onto the fibular head in conjunction with the distal tendon of biceps femoris; and the popliteus tendon, which attaches to the popliteal notch of the lateral femur.

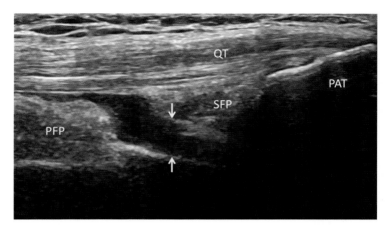

Longitudinal view of the suprapatellar pouch (arrows) with a normal volume of fluid and distal quadriceps tendon (QT) as it attaches to the patella (PAT) at 30° of knee flexion. The suprapatellar fat pad (SFP) and pre-femoral fat pad (PFP) lie on either side of the suprapatellar pouch.

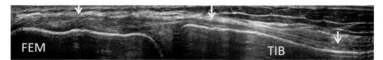

Longitudinal view of the medial collateral ligament (arrows) attaching to the medial epicondyle of the femur (FEM) and medial tibial metaphysis (TIB).

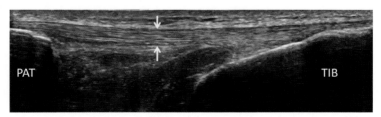

Longitudinal view of the patella tendon (arrows) and its attachments onto the patella (PAT) and tibia (TIB).

MEASUREMENTS

Suprapatella pouch thickness (at 30° of knee flexion)	4 mm	
Medial collateral ligament thickness	**Proximal**	**Distal**
	5 mm	3 mm
Distal quadriceps tendon thickness (mean ± SD)	**Males**	**Females**
	5.1 ± 0.6 mm	4.9 ± 0.6 mm
Mid-patellar tendon thickness (mean ± SD)	**Males**	**Females**
	3.1 ± 0.4 mm	2.9 ± 0.5 mm
Iliotibial band thickness (mean ± SD)	**Femoral condyle**	**Tibial condyle**
	1.95 mm ± 0.3 mm	3.4 mm ± 0.5 mm

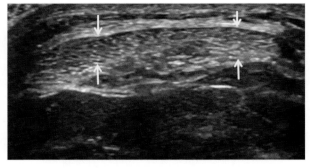

Transverse view of the mid-patella tendon (arrows).

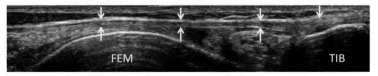

Longitudinal view of the ilio-tibial band (arrows) as it attaches onto the antero-lateral tibia. (FEM, femur; TIB, tibia)

FURTHER READING

Goh LA, Chhem RK, Wang SC, Chee T. Iliotibial band thickness: Sonographic measurements in asymptomatic volunteers. *J Clin Ultrasound*. 2003; 31:239–244.

Morris-Stiff G, Haynes M, Ogunbiyi S, Townsend E, Shetty S, Winter RK, Lewis MH. Is assessment of popliteal artery diameter in patients undergoing screening for abdominal aortic aneurysms a worthwhile procedure? *Eur J Vasc Endovasc Surg*. 2005; 30:71–74.

Schmidt WA, Schmidt H, Schicke B, Gromnica-Ihle E. Standard reference values for musculoskeletal ultrasonography. *Ann Rheum Dis*. 2004; 63:988–994.

Posterior knee

PREPARATION
None.

POSITION
Prone with the knee extended for assessment of the popliteal fossa.

TRANSDUCER
7.0–15.0 MHz linear transducer.

METHOD
The popliteal vessels and any cysts around the knee are evaluated in axial and longitudinal planes. Doppler and color flow are used to assess the popliteal vessels.

APPEARANCE
The popliteal artery and vein are aligned in a sagittal oblique plane in the popliteal fossa, between the medial and lateral head of gastrocnemius, and appear as anechoic tubular structures with echogenic walls.

FURTHER READING

Goh LA, Chhem RK, Wang SC, Chee T. Iliotibial band thickness: Sonographic measurements in asymptomatic volunteers. *J Clin Ultrasound.* 2003; 31:239–244.

Morris-Stiff G, Haynes M, Ogunbiyi S, Townsend E, Shetty S, Winter RK, Lewis MH. Is assessment of popliteal artery diameter in patients undergoing screening for abdominal aortic aneurysms a worthwhile procedure? *Eur J Vasc Endovasc Surg.* 2005; 30:71–74.

Schmidt WA, Schmidt H, Schicke B, Gromnica-Ihle E. Standard reference values for musculoskeletal ultrasonography. *Ann Rheum Dis.* 2004; 63:988–994.

LOWER LIMB: ANKLE

Anterior, medial, and lateral tendons

PREPARATION
None.

POSITION
Supine.

TRANSDUCER
10.0–15.0 MHz linear transducer.

METHOD
With the patient supine, the transducer is placed longitudinally across the tibiotalar joint to assess for fluid in the anterior recess.

APPEARANCE

	Probe position	Appearance
Medial	Transverse image at the medial ankle. Each tendon assessed in transverse and longitudinal section.	Tibialis posterior is identified just behind the malleolus, and flexor digitorum longus lies just posterior to this. Flexor hallucis longus lies deep and may be more readily identified by a posterior approach.
Anterior	Anterior to the tibiotalar joint	Tibialis anterior, extensor hallucis longus, and extensor digitorum longus (medial to lateral).
Lateral	Transverse behind the lateral malleolus	Peroneus brevis and longus tendons. Peroneus brevis lies anteromedially to longus and can be followed to its insertion at the base of the 5th metatarsal, while peroneus longus crosses the sole to insert at the base of the 1st metatarsal and the medial cuneiform.

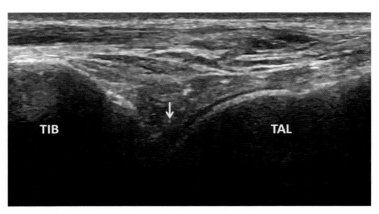

Longitudinal view through the anterior joint space of the ankle (TIB, tibia; TAL, talus). The arrow points to the anterior synovial recess, where the joint may be evaluated for the presence of an effusion.

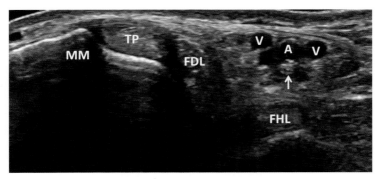

Transverse view of the medial ankle tendons behind the medial malleolus (MM). (TP, tibialis posterior; FDL, flexor digitorum longus; FHL, flexor hallucis longus.) Posterior tibial artery (A), veins (V), and posterior tibial nerve (arrow) are also demonstrated.

MEASUREMENTS

The anterior recess of the tibiotalar joint may normally contain up to 3 mm depth of fluid. Fluid may normally be identified in the tibialis posterior tendon sheath at, or below, the malleolar level, within the peroneal tendons below the malleolar level, and may be asymmetric. The flexor digitorum longus and flexor hallucis longus may also normally show a small amount of surrounding fluid, unlike the anterior tendons, which normally do not.

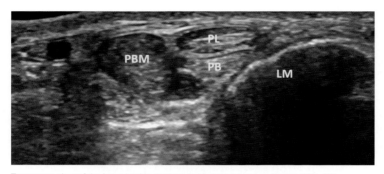

Transverse view of the lateral ankle tendons behind the lateral malleolus (LM). (PB, peroneus brevis tendon; PBM peroneus brevis muscle; PL, peroneus longus tendon.)

The tibialis posterior is the largest of the medial tendons, measuring 4–6 mm in diameter. It may be followed to its insertion into the navicular where the fibers normally fan out.

FURTHER READING

Bianchi S, Martinoli C, Gaignot C, De Gautard R, Meyer JM. Ultrasound of the ankle: Anatomy of the tendons, bursae, and ligaments. *Semin Musculoskelet Radiol.* 2005; 9:243–259.

Nazarian LN, Nandkumar MR, Martin CE, Schweitzer ME. Synovial fluid in the hindfoot and ankle: Detection of amount and distribution with US. *Radiology.* 1995; 197:275–278.

Schmidt WA, Schmidt H, Schicke B, Gromnica-Ihle E. Standard reference values for musculoskeletal ultrasonography. *Ann Rheum Dis.* 2004; 63:988–994.

Achilles tendon

PREPARATION
None.

POSITION
The patient is prone with feet hanging over the edge of the examination couch or supine with hip flexed and externally rotated and the knee flexed.

TRANSDUCER
10.0–15.0 MHz linear transducer.

METHOD
The transducer is placed over the Achilles tendon longitudinally and transversely to assess the full length of the tendon from the musculo-tendinous junction to calcaneal insertion. Movement of the ankle is helpful to fully evaluate tears.

APPEARANCE
The Achilles tendon has an ovoid shape in transverse section. The calcaneal insertion of the tendon may appear of low reflectivity due to anisotropy or the presence of cartilage at the enthesis. The plantaris tendon should be separately identified as it runs from the posterolateral knee to insert on the posteromedial calcaneus/Achilles. The retrocalcaneal bursa lies between the Achilles tendon and the calcaneus.

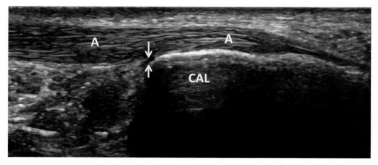

Longitudinal view of the distal Achilles tendon (A) attaching onto the calcaneum (CAL). The hypoechoic retrocalcaneal bursa (arrows) lies between the Achilles tendon and calcaneum.

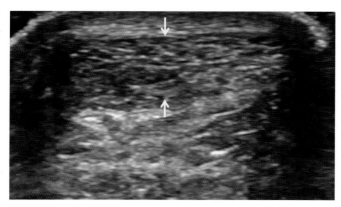

Achilles tendon (arrows) in transverse view at the level of the medial malleolus where its thickness can be measured.

MEASUREMENTS

Retrocalcaneal bursa	Up to 3 mm depth of fluid
Achilles tendon thickness at the level of the medial malleolus in transverse section	5.3 mm (range 4–6 mm)

FURTHER READING

Fornage BD. Achilles tendon: US examination. *Radiology*. 1986; 159:759–764.

Nazarian LN, Nandkumar MR, Martin CE, Schweitzer ME. Synovial fluid in the hindfoot and ankle: Detection of amount and distribution with US. *Radiology*. 1995; 197:275–278.

Schmidt WA, Schmidt H, Schicke B, Gromnica-Ihle E. Standard reference values for musculoskeletal ultrasonography. *Ann Rheum Dis*. 2004; 63:988–994.

LOWER LIMB: FOOT

Plantar fascia

PREPARATION
None.

POSITION
Prone with feet hanging over the edge of the examination couch or supine with the hip flexed and externally rotated and the knee flexed.

TRANSDUCER
7.0–10.0 MHz linear array transducer.

METHOD
The transducer is placed longitudinally and transversely across the plantar fascia. The origin of the central portion of the fascia is at the calcaneal tuberosity, and the fascia is traced to the mid-arch but becomes superficial and thin in the forefoot. Look for evidence of a subcalcaneal spur.

APPEARANCE
The plantar fascia is well defined and of moderately high reflectivity with a uniform fibrillary pattern, but may show low reflectivity at the calcaneal tuberosity due to anisotropy.

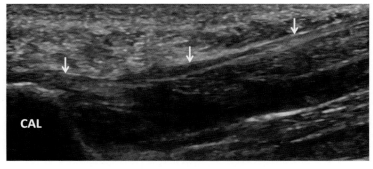

Longitudinal view of the plantar fascia (arrows) across the sole of the foot (CAL, calcaneal tuberosity).

MEASUREMENTS

Thicknesses of the proximal plantar fascia measurements are taken in the longitudinal plane close to the calcaneal attachment. A plantar fascia thickness of up to 4 mm is considered within normal limits.

FURTHER READING

McMillan AM, Landorf KB, Barrett JT, Menz HB, Bird AR. Diagnostic imaging for chronic plantar heel pain: A systematic review and meta-analysis. *J Foot Ankle Res.* 2009; 2:32.

INTERDIGITAL WEB SPACES

PREPARATION
None.

POSITION
Supine.

TRANSDUCER
7.0–10.0 MHz linear array transducer.

METHOD
The transducer is placed transversely across the dorsum of the foot to examine the spaces between the metatarsal heads. At the same time finger pressure is applied to the plantar surface of web space under examination. Alternatively, forced flexion of the toes or squeezing of the metatarsal heads together by pressure from the examiner's hand may displace a neuroma for improved visualization. The process is repeated with the probe on the plantar surface and finger pressure on the dorsum of the foot. The interdigital space is also examined in longitudinal section by aligning the probe within the web space.

APPEARANCE
The normal interspace appears as high-reflective fat bounded by the high-reflective metatarsal cortex on each side. A Morton's neuroma appears as a noncompressible low-reflective mass, while a bursa appears as a compressible low-reflective mass.

FURTHER READING
Redd RA, Peters VJ, Emery SF, Branch HM, Rifkin MD.
   Morton neuroma: Sonographic evaluation. *Radiology*. 1989;
   171:415–417.

Pediatric and Neonatal

10

UPPER ABDOMEN

Annamaria Deganello, Maria E. Sellars, and Paul S. Sidhu

Liver (pediatric)

PREPARATION
None.

POSITION
Supine, right anterior oblique positions to demonstrate the porta hepatis.

TRANSDUCER
4.0–9.0 MHz curvilinear transducer.

METHOD
Longitudinal images of the right lobe are taken in the midclavicular and midline positions. The length of the liver is measured from the uppermost portion of the dome of the diaphragm to the inferior tip.

APPEARANCE
Uniform pattern of medium-strength echoes.

MEASUREMENTS

Length of right lobe of liver versus age	
Age range (months)	**Mean ± SD (mm)**
1–3	64 ± 10.4
4–6	73 ± 10.8
7–9	79 ± 8.0
12–30	85 ± 10.0
36–59	86 ± 11.8
60–83	100 ± 13.6
84–107	105 ± 10.6
108–131	105 ± 12.5
132–155	115 ± 14.0
156–179	118 ± 14.6
180–200	121 ± 11.7

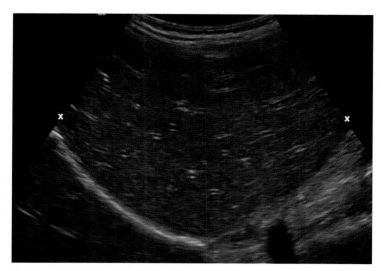

The length of the right lobe of the liver is obtained in the longitudinal plane in the midclavicular line (cursors).

Length of right lobe of liver versus body weight	
Weight (kg)	Mean ± SD (mm)
20	105 ± 14
30	112 ± 13
40	116 ± 12
50	119 ± 15
60	123 ± 14

FURTHER READING

Konus OL, Ozdemir A, Akkaya A, Erbas G, Celik H, Isik S. Normal liver, spleen, and kidney dimensions in neonates, infants, and children: Evaluation with sonography. *AJR Am J Roentgenol.* 1998; 171:1693–1698.

Safak AA, Simsek E, Bahcebasi T. Sonographic assessment of the normal limits and percentile curves of liver, spleen, and kidney dimensions in healthy school-aged children. *J Ultrasound Med.* 2005; 24:1359–1364.

Gallbladder (neonatal)

PREPARATION
Patient should fast prior to the examination.

POSITION
The gallbladder is initially examined in the supine position and may be turned to right anterior oblique position.

TRANSDUCER
8.0–14.0 MHz linear transducer.

METHOD
Longitudinal and transverse images are obtained from a subcostal or intercostal approach on deep inspiration in the supine and right anterior oblique positions.

APPEARANCE
On a longitudinal image the gallbladder appears as an echo-free, pear-shaped structure. The gallbladder wall is smooth and is seen as a line of high reflectivity.

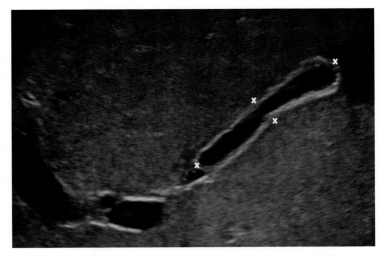

Longitudinal image through the gallbladder with length and depth measurements in a 2-week-old child (between cursors).

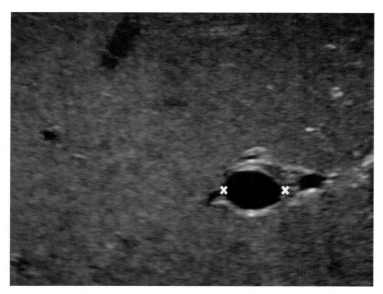

Transverse image from a subcostal approach on deep inspiration demonstrating the measurement of width in a 2-week-old child (between cursors).

MEASUREMENTS

Newborn	Length	Width
	30–32 mm	1/3 of length

FURTHER READING

Carroll BA, Oppenheimer DA, Muller HH. High-frequency real-time ultrasound of the neonatal biliary system. *Radiology*. 1982; 145:437–440.

Gallbladder (pediatric)

PREPARATION
Younger patients should fast for 3 hours; older children should fast for 6–8 hours prior to the examination.

POSITION
The gallbladder is initially examined in the supine position, and then the patient is turned to right anterior oblique position.

TRANSDUCER
4.0–6.0 MHz curvilinear transducer.

METHOD
Longitudinal and transverse images are obtained from a subcostal or intercostal approach in the supine and right anterior oblique positions.

APPEARANCE
On a longitudinal image the gallbladder appears as an echo-free, pear-shaped structure.

MEASUREMENTS

Age (years)	Length Mean ± SD (cm)	Width Mean ± SD (cm)	Volume Mean ± SD (cc)
<1	3.3 (± 0.8)	0.9 (± 0.4)	1.8 (± 1.7)
1	4.2 (± 0.6)	1.4 (± 0.3)	4.6 (± 2.6)
2	4.5 (± 0.6)	1.5 (± 0.3)	5.9 (± 2.4)
3	4.3 (± 0.6)	1.5 (± 0.2)	4.9 (± 1.7)
4	4.7 (± 1.3)	1.5 (± 0.3)	5.9 (± 2.6)
5	5.0 (± 1.0)	1.7 (± 0.4)	7.8 (± 4.8)
6	4.9 (± 1.0)	1.6 (± 0.3)	7.0 (± 3.6)
7	5.1 (± 0.9)	1.6 (± 0.4)	7.2 (± 3.8)
8	5.3 (± 1.0)	1.7 (± 0.4)	8.5 (± 4.8)
9	5.5 (± 1.0)	1.8 (± 0.5)	10.0 (± 5.9)
10	5.6 (± 0.8)	1.9 (± 0.4)	11.5 (± 5.3)
11	6.0 (± 1.0)	1.9 (± 0.4)	12.6 (± 6.6)

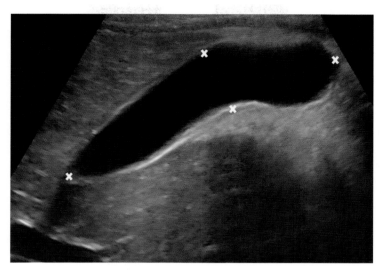

Longitudinal image through the gallbladder of a 5-year-old child with length and depth measurements (between cursors).

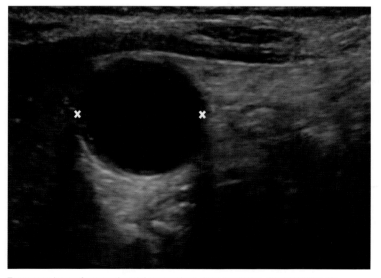

Transverse image from a subcostal approach on deep inspiration demonstrating the measurement of width (between cursors).

Age (years)	Length Mean ± SD (cm)	Width Mean ± SD (cm)	Volume Mean ± SD (cc)
12	6.1 (±0.8)	1.8 (± 0.6)	12.1 (± 7.8)
13	6.6 (±1.3)	1.9 (± 0.6)	14.0 (± 8.4)
14	6.8 (±1.1)	2.0 (± 0.6)	15.2 (± 8.1)
15	6.3 (± 1.3)	1.9 (± 0.6)	13.3 (± 9.5)
16	5.9 (± 1.1)	1.9 (± 0.6)	11.9 (± 6.6)

FURTHER READING

McGahan JP, Phillips HE, Cox KL. Sonography of the normal pediatric gallbladder and biliary tract. *Radiology.* 1982; 144:873–875.

Yoo JH, Kwak HJ, Lee MJ, Suh JS, Rhee CS. Sonographic measurements of normal gallbladder sizes in children. *J Clin Ultrasound.* 2003; 31:80–84.

Common bile duct (pediatric)

PREPARATION
None.

POSITION
Initially supine, then turn to the right anterior oblique position to demonstrate the common duct.

TRANSDUCER
4.0–6.0 MHz curvilinear transducer.

METHOD
Patient is imaged in a subcostal position in the longitudinal plane or from an intercostal position. The common bile duct may be identified by means of the anatomic course within the gastroduodenal ligament, coursing distally to the head of the pancreas and absence of flow with Doppler interrogation. The internal diameter of the extrahepatic duct is measured from inner wall to inner wall.

APPEARANCE
With high-resolution imaging, normal intrahepatic ducts can be visualized as tubular structures with thin high-reflective walls. The term *common duct* is used, because it is not possible to demonstrate the entrance of the cystic duct on an ultrasound, and thus be able to differentiate the common hepatic duct from the common bile duct.

MEASUREMENTS
The common duct of neonates and children younger than 1 year should be 1.6 mm or less in inner wall to inner wall diameter. The size increases slowly with age. The common duct during childhood and early adolescence should not measure more than 2.5–3.0 mm in diameter. It is a distensible structure that demonstrates small but statistically significant changes in size during daily fluctuations in the bile flow.

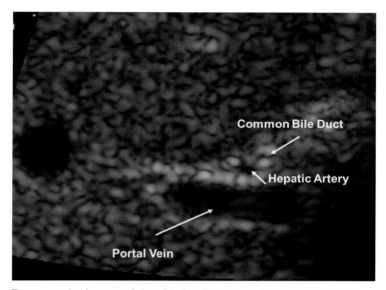

The common duct is measured at a point where it passes anterior to the right portal vein with the hepatic artery seen in cross section between the duct and the vein.

Diameter of common bile duct in children according to age (in a Chinese population)			
Age (years)	Minimum size (mm)	Maximum size (mm)	Mean ± SD (mm)
0–1	0.40	3.2	1.15 (± 0.53)
1–4	0.80	4.00	1.69 (± 0.55)
4–7	0.80	3.50	1.73 (± 0.56)
7–14	1.40	4.40	2.36 (± 0.79)

FURTHER READING

Hernanz–Schulman M, Ambrosino MM, Freeman PC, Quinn CB. Common bile duct in children. Sonographic dimensions. *Radiology.* 1995; 195:193–195.

Zhang Y, Wang KL, Li SX, Bai YZ, Ren WD, Xie LM, Zhang SC. Ultrasonographic dimensions of the common bile duct in Chinese children: Results of 343 cases. *J Pediatr Surg.* 2013; 48:1892–1896.

Spleen (pediatric)

PREPARATION
None.

POSITION
Left upper abdomen in the mid-axillary line, then turn patient to the left anterior oblique position as necessary to view the spleen.

TRANSDUCER
2.0–6.0 MHz curvilinear transducer.

METHOD
Splenic length is measured during quiet breathing, obtained from a coronal plane that includes the hilum. The greatest longitudinal distance between the splenic dome and the tip (splenic length) is measured. Transverse, longitudinal, and diagonal diameters can be measured from the image showing the maximum cross-sectional area in a coronal plane.

APPEARANCE
The spleen should show a uniform echo pattern. It is slightly less reflective than the liver.

MEASUREMENTS
Measurement of length: A measurement of length and diameter can be made in the oblique plane at the 10th and 11th intercostal space, through the splenic hilum.

Length of spleen versus body weight	
Weight (kg)	**Mean $\pm$ SD (mm)**
20	78 ± 9
30	80 ± 9
40	83 ± 18
50	86 ± 13
60	91 ± 12

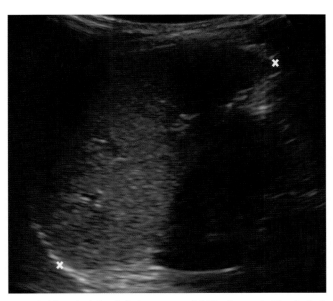

Measurement of the splenic length (between cursors), taking the greatest longitudinal distance between the splenic dome and the tip of the spleen.

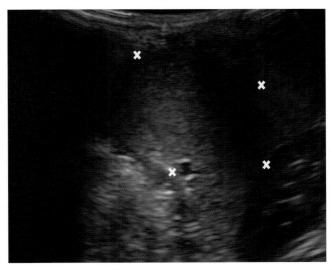

Two further measurements are obtained to calculate the splenic area (between cursors).

Spleen length versus age and sex		
Age range in months (m) and years (y)	Male mean ± SD (mm)	Female mean ± SD (mm)
0–3 m	4.6 ± 0.84	4.4 ± 0.57
3–6 m	5.8 ± 0.65	5.2 ± 0.47
6–12 m	6.4 ± 0.78	6.3 ± 0.68
1–2 y	6.8 ± 0.72	6.3 ± 0.69
2–4 y	7.6 ± 1.07	7.5 ± 0.83
4–6 y	8.1± 1.01	8.0 ± 0.74
6–8 y	8.9 ± 0.91	8.2 ± 0.99
8–10 y	9.0 ± 1.02	8.7 ± 0.92
10–12 y	9.8 ± 1.05	9.1 ± 1.09
12–14 y	10.2 ± 0.81	9.8 ± 1.02
14–17 y	10.7 ± 0.90	10.3 ± 0.69

Measurement of area: View the spleen in the longitudinal axis, in deep inspiration. The interface between the lung and spleen serves as the transverse diameter, and the longitudinal diameter is measured from here to the splenic tip. The diagonal diameter is measured from this lateral spleen–lung interface to the medial spleen margin. The cross-sectional area is calculated as follows:

$$\frac{\text{Diagonal}}{\sqrt{(\text{Transverse}^2 + \text{Longitudinal}^2)/2}}$$

Normal	Diameter in cm (mean ± SD)
Transverse diameter	5.5 ± 1.4
Longitudinal diameter	5.8 ± 1.8
Diagonal diameter	3.7 ± 1.0

FURTHER READING

Megremis SD, Vlachonikolis IG, Tsilimigaki AM. Spleen length in childhood with US: Normal values based on age, sex, and somatometric parameters. *Radiology*. 2004; 231:129–134.

Niederau C, Sonnenberg A, Muller JE, Erckenbrecht JF, Scholten T, Fritsch WP. Sonographic measurements of the normal liver, spleen, pancreas, and portal vein. *Radiology*. 1983; 149:537–540.

Safak AA, Simsek E, Bahcebasi T. Sonographic assessment of the normal limits and percentile curves of liver, spleen, and kidney dimensions in healthy school-aged children. *J Ultrasound Med*. 2005; 24:1359–1364.

Pancreas (pediatric)

PREPARATION
None.

POSITION
Supine, decubitus, and semi-decubitus positions with the left side elevated.

TRANSDUCER
5.0–7.5 MHz curvilinear transducer.

METHOD
Maximum anteroposterior diameters of the head, body, and tail of the pancreas are measured on transverse/oblique images.

APPEARANCE
The pancreas should be homogenous with a reflectivity equal to or slightly greater than that of the adjacent liver. The pancreatic duct may be seen as a single high-reflective line and usually measures less than 1 mm.

MEASUREMENTS

Normal dimensions of the pancreas as a function of age			
	Maximum anteroposterior dimensions ± SD (cm)		
Patient age	Head	Body	Tail
<1 month	1.0 ± 0.4	0.6 ± 0.2	1.0 ± 0.04
1 month–1 year	1.5 ± 0.5	0.8 ± 0.3	1.2 ± 0.4
1–5 years	1.7 ± 0.3	1.0 ± 0.2	1.8 ± 0.4
5–10 years	1.6 ± 0.4	1.0 ± 0.3	1.8 ± 0.4
10–19 years	1.0 ± 0.5	1.1 ± 0.3	2.0 ± 0.4

FURTHER READING
Siegel MJ, Martin KW, Worthington JL. Normal and abnormal pancreas in children. *Radiology*. 1987; 165:15–18.

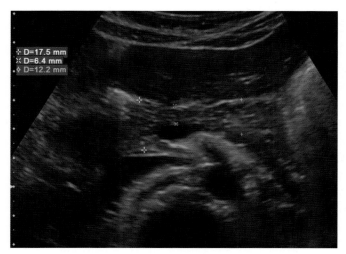

Transverse image through the pancreas at the level of the confluence of the splenic vein and the superior mesenteric vein, in a 12-year-old male subject. The three cursors measure the anteroposterior diameters of the head, body, and tail.

Adrenal glands (neonatal)

PREPARATION
None.

POSITION
Supine.

TRANSDUCER
6.0–7.5 MHz curvilinear transducer.

METHOD
Image from flanks in sagittal, coronal, and transverse planes.

APPEARANCE
The adrenals have an oval shape in the transverse plane and an inverted Y-shape in the longitudinal plane. A rim of low reflectivity surrounds the thin high-reflective core. The right gland is seen in 97% and the left gland in 83%.

MEASUREMENTS
Length is measured as maximum cephalocaudal dimension, from the apex to the base of the gland. The maximum transverse and antero-posterior diameters are measured in a transverse plane perpendicular to the length of one of the wings.

Length of the adrenal glands versus gestational age	
Gestational age (weeks)	**Mean ± SD (mm)**
16	4.2 ± 0.70
17	4.6 ± 0.70
18	5.0 ± 0.70
19	5.4 ± 0.70
20	5.8 ± 0.70
21	6.2 ± 0.70
22	6.6 ± 0.70
23	6.9 ± 0.71
24	7.3 ± 0.71

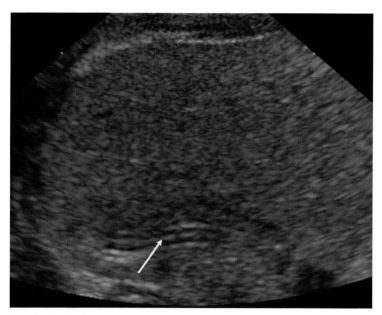

The adrenal gland is represented by a thin echogenic core (arrow) surrounded by an echo-poor rim. Length is measured as a maximum cephalocaudal dimension, and the width is the maximum dimension perpendicular to the length of one of the wings.

Length of the adrenal glands versus gestational age	
Gestational age (weeks)	Mean ± SD (mm)
25	7.6 ± 0.71
26	8.0 ± 0.71
27	8.3 ± 0.72
28	8.6 ± 0.72
29	8.9 ± 0.72
30	9.1 ± 0.73
31	9.4 ± 0.73
32	9.7 ± 0.73
33	9.9 ± 0.74

Length of the adrenal glands versus gestational age	
Gestational age (weeks)	Mean ± SD (mm)
34	10.2 ± 0.74
35	10.4 ± 0.75
36	10.6 ± 0.75
37	10.8 ± 0.76
38	11.0 ± 0.76
39	11.2 ± 0.77
40	11.3 ± 0.77
41	11.5 ± 0.78

The size of the adrenal gland diminishes rapidly in the first 6 weeks of post-natal life.

FURTHER READING

Oppenheimer DA, Carroll BA, Yousem S. Sonography of the normal neonatal adrenal gland. *Radiology*. 1983; 146:157–160.

van Vuuren SH, Damen-Elias HA, Stigter RH, van der Doef R, Goldschmeding R, de Jong TP, Westers P, Visser GH, Pistorius LR. Size and volume charts of fetal kidney, renal pelvis and adrenal gland. *Ultrasound Obstet Gynecol*. 2012; 40:659–664.

Adrenal glands (infant)

PREPARATION
None.

POSITION
Supine.

TRANSDUCER
6.0–7.5 MHz curvilinear transducer.

METHOD
Image from flanks in sagittal, coronal, and transverse planes.

APPEARANCE
Thin high-reflective core representing the cortex, surrounded by a rim of low reflectivity representing the medulla. As the infant grows, at 2 months, the cortex gets smaller and the medulla larger in proportion. At 5–6 months the whole gland is smaller, and generally of high reflectivity. At the age of 12 months, the gland is similar to the adult gland and becomes low-reflective.

MEASUREMENTS
Length is measured as maximum cephalocaudal dimension, from the apex to the base of the gland. The maximum transverse and antero-posterior diameters are measured in a transverse plane perpendicular to the length of one of the wings.

Mean (± SD) serial adrenal measurements (mm) in neonates			
Day	**Transverse**	**Anteroposterior**	**Length**
1	17.9 (± 2.7)	9.6 (± 2.1)	17.3 (± 1.8)
3	14.8 (± 3.3)	7.5 (± 2.2)	12.8 (± 3.2)
5	13.7 (± 2.1)	6.9 (± 1.6)	11.4 (± 2.7)
11	11.8 (± 2.5)	5.9 (± 1.4)	8.9 (± 2.0)
21	10.8 (± 1.9)	5.6 (± 0.5)	8.2 (± 1.2)
42	|9.5 (± 1.5)	5.7 (± 1.0)	7.7 (± 0.9)

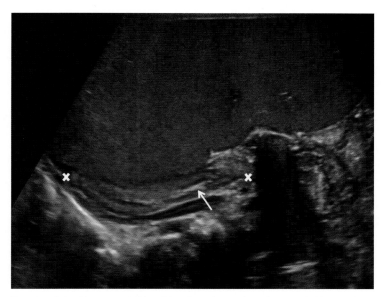

The adrenal gland is represented by a thin echogenic core (arrow) surrounded by an echo-poor rim. Length is measured as a maximum cephalocaudal dimension (between cursors), and the width is the maximum dimension perpendicular to the length of one of the wings.

FURTHER READING

Scott EM, Thomas A, McGarrigle HH, Lachelin GC. Serial adrenal ultrasonography in normal neonates. *J Ultrasound Med*. 1990; 9:279–283.

Pyloric stenosis

PREPARATION

No food for at least 2 hours prior to the examination.

POSITION

Supine or right anterior oblique.

TRANSDUCER

5.0–8.0 MHz curvilinear transducer or a 7.0–10.0 MHz linear transducer.

METHOD

Longitudinal and transverse preliminary views right of midline at the level of subxiphoid space. The infant is usually bottle fed at the time of the examination. Image with patient right side down and obtain longitudinal and transverse views as before.

APPEARANCE

Thickened muscle is seen as a low-reflective layer, superficial to the high-reflective mucosal layer. In the transverse plane, the canal resembles a "doughnut," medial to the gallbladder and anterior to the right kidney. There is an absence of peristalsis distally, whereas the stomach is distended and shows visible peristaltic wave.

MEASUREMENTS

Pyloric length (b) = ≥ 14 mm

Pyloric muscle thickness (c) = ≥ 3 mm

FURTHER READING

Haller JO, Cohen HL. Hypertrophic pyloric stenosis: Diagnosis using US. *Radiology*. 1986; 161:335–339.

Hernanz-Schulman M. Pyloric stenosis: Role of imaging. *Pediatr Radiol*. 2009; 39:S134–9.

Hernanz-Schulman M, Sells LL, Ambrosino MM, Heller RM, Stein SM, Neblett WW III. Hypertrophic pyloric stenosis in the infant without a palpable olive: Accuracy of sonographic diagnosis. *Radiology*. 1994; 193:771–776.

O'Keeffe FN, Stansberry SD, Swischuk LE, Hayden CK Jr. Antropyloric muscle thickness at US in infants: What is normal? *Radiology*. 1991; 178:827–830.

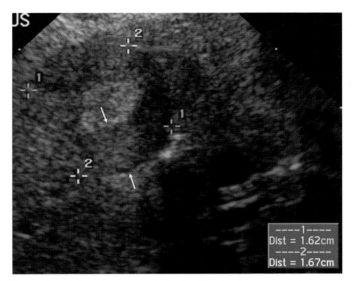

Axial image through the pylorus demonstrating the "doughnut" appearance (between cursors); the low echogenic muscle layer is seen (between arrows).

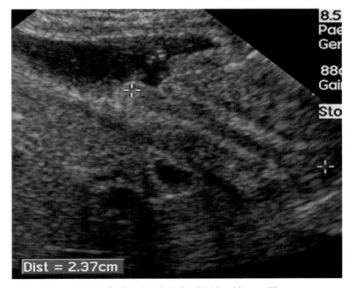

Longitudinal measurement of pyloric length in the right decubitus position.

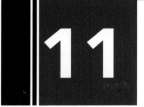

11

RENAL TRACT

*Annamaria Deganello and
Maria E. Sellars*

Renal size (pediatric)

PREPARATION
None.

POSITION
The prone position is useful in children.

TRANSDUCER
4.0–6.0 MHz curvilinear transducer.

METHOD
Image the right kidney using the liver as an acoustic window. The left kidney is usually more difficult to visualize. The left anterior oblique 45° or right decubitus position may help. Both kidneys must be imaged in both longitudinal and transverse planes.

APPEARANCE
The reflectivity of the renal cortex is less than that of the adjacent liver and spleen. The renal capsule can be identified as a thin, high-reflective rim. The renal pyramids are poorly defined structures seen at the outer edge of the renal sinus. The renal sinus contains multiple structures—the pelvis, calyces, vessels, and fat—and is usually of high reflectivity.

MEASUREMENTS
Measurements of renal size are taken in the maximum longitudinal plane. In children, the length of the kidneys correlates best to height, although charts against age and weight are available. Differences between the left and right kidney are minimal.

Renal lengths related to body height		
Body height (cm)	**Right kidney mean ± SD (cm)**	**Left kidney mean ± SD (cm)**
48–64	5.0 ± 0.58	5.0 ± 0.55
54–73	5.3 ± 0.53	5.6 ± 0.55
65–78	5.9 ± 0.52	6.1 ± 0.46
71–92	6.1 ± 0.34	6.6 ± 0.53
85–109	6.7 ± 0.51	7.1 ± 0.45

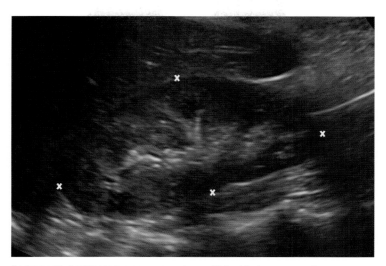

On the longitudinal image two measurements are obtained (between cursors).

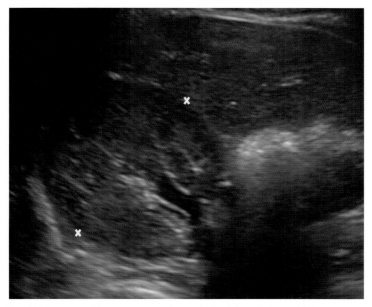

The width is measured from a transverse image obtained through the renal hilum (between cursors).

Renal lengths related to body height		
Body height (cm)	Right kidney mean ± SD (cm)	Left kidney mean ± SD (cm)
100–130	7.4 ± 0.55	7.9 ± 0.59
110–131	8.0 ± 0.66	8.4 ± 0.66
124–149	8.0 ± 0.70	8.4 ± 0.74
137–153	8.9 ± 0.62	9.1 ± 0.84
143–168	9.4 ± 0.59	9.6 ± 0.89
152–175	9.2 ± 0.70	9.9 ± 0.75

Length of the right kidney versus body weight	
Weight (kg)	Mean ± SD (mm)
20	81 ± 8
30	87 ± 7
40	89 ± 6
50	83 ± 8
60	98 ± 7

Length of the left kidney versus body weight	
Weight (kg)	Mean ± SD (mm)
20	83 ± 8
30	86 ± 8
40	90 ± 8
50	93 ± 9
60	98 ± 9

Adapted from Dinkel et al. 1985, Rosenbaum et al. 1984, Konus et al. 1998.

FURTHER READING

Dinkel E, Erkel M, Dittrich M, Peters H, Berres M, Schulte-Wissermann H. Kidney size in childhood. Sonographical growth charts for kidney length and volume. *Pediatr Radiol.* 1985; 15:38–43.

Konus OL, Ozdemir A, Akkaya A, Erbas G, Celik H, Isik S. Normal liver, spleen, and kidney dimensions in neonates, infants, and children: Evaluation with sonography. *AJR Am J Roentgenol.* 1998; 171:1693–1698.

Rosenbaum DM, Korngold E, Teele RL. Sonographic assessment of renal length in normal children. *AJR Am J Roentgenol.* 1984; 142:467–469.

Safak AA, Simsek E, Bahcebasi T. Sonographic assessment of the normal limits and percentile curves of liver, spleen, and kidney dimensions in healthy school-aged children. *J Ultrasound Med.* 2005; 24:1359–1364.

Renal size (neonates and infants)

PREPARATION
None.

POSITION
Supine.

TRANSDUCER
5.0–8.0 MHz curvilinear transducer and 9.0 MHz linear transducer.

METHOD
Image the right kidney using the liver as an acoustic window. The left kidney is usually more difficult to visualize. The left anterior oblique 45° or right decubitus position may help. Both kidneys must be imaged in both longitudinal and transverse planes.

APPEARANCE
Accentuated corticomedullary differentiation is a normal finding in neonates and infants (age 1 day–6 months). The medullary pyramids are seen as low-reflective triangles arranged in the circular fashion around the central echogenic renal sinus, while the renal cortex has higher reflectivity.

MEASUREMENTS

Renal lengths in term newborn infants		
Renal length	Male mean ± SD (mm)	Female mm mean ± SD (mm)
Right kidney longitudinal	42.6 ± 3.2	41.5 ± 3.5
Right kidney anteroposterior	20.2 ± 1.8	19.6 ± 1.6
Left kidney longitudinal	44.0 ± 3.3	42.2 ± 3.4
Left kidney anteroposterior	21.5 ± 1.8	20.8 ± 1.7

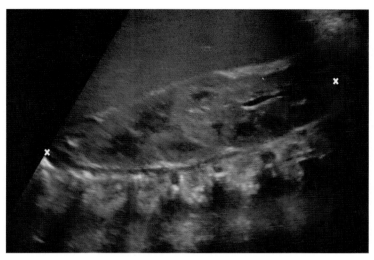

On the longitudinal image two measurements are obtained (between cursors).

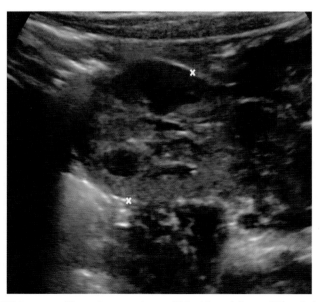

The width is measured from a transverse image obtained through the renal hilum (between cursors).

Renal lengths in preterm newborn infants according to weight

Kidney	Gender	Weight (g)	Renal length (range in mm)
Right kidney longitudinal	Female	≤ 750	23.7–41.0
		751–1000	25.2–40.5
		1001–1250	28.2–45.8
		1251–1500	28.4–44.2
		1501–1750	32.2–43.4
		1751–2000	32.3–49.3
		2001–2250	35.2–48.1
		2251–2500	35.3–48.1
		≥ 2501	37.3–47.9
	Male	≤ 750	23.0–37.3
		751–1000	25.0–39.7
		1001–1250	28.5–41.0
		1251–1500	25.4–48.4
		1501–1750	31.0–49.7
		1751–2000	30.8–50.2
		2001–2250	33.0–56.0
		2251–2500	36.0–51.0
		≥ 2501	38.7–54.5
Right kidney anteroposterior	Female	≤ 750	11.1–17.1
		751–1000	10.8–19.1
		1001–1250	11.9–21.7
		1251–1500	12.8–25.6
		1501–1750	13.9–24.8
		1751–2000	13.4–22.4
		2001–2250	15.0–24.1
		2251–2500	15.2–23.1
		≥ 2501	13.7–23.7
	Male	≤ 750	9.7–16.2
		751–1000	9.7–22.0
		1001–1250	10.3–20.7
		1251–1500	9.5–22.4
		1501–1750	12.0–19.4
		1751–2000	13.0–23.1
		2001–2250	13.9–25.5
		2251–2500	13.3–24.4
		≥ 2501	14.9–30.5

Renal lengths in preterm newborn infants according to weight

Kidney	Gender	Weight (g)	Renal length (range in mm)
Left kidney longitudinal	Female	≤ 750	21.4–37.6
		751–1000	25.5–37.8
		1001–1250	27.4–42.9
		1251–1500	29.3–44.3
		1501–1750	31.8–46.8
		1751–2000	32.6–47.5
		2001–2250	35.9–46.8
		2251–2500	35.2–50.0
		≥ 2501	38.7–50.3
	Male	≤ 750	26.7–33.6
		751–1000	24.1–39.9
		1001–1250	28.3–45.1
		1251–1500	23.8–46.1
		1501–1750	30.5–54.0
		1751–2000	30.9–49.7
		2001–2250	33.6–52.2
		2251–250	36.2–48.4
		≥ 2501	39.9–52.4
Left kidney anteroposterior	Female	≤ 750	10.1–16.4
		751–1000	10.3–18.2
		1001–1250	10.2–22.2
		1251–1500	13.4–21.1
		1501–1750	12.0–20.5
		1751–2000	13.0–21.6
		2001–2250	12.5–21.9
		2251–2500	13.6–26.1
		≥ 2501	14.0–22.5
	Male	≤ 750	11.1–16.0
		751–1000	9.6–21.5
		1001–1250	10.3–20.3
		1251–1500	11.3–21.9
		1501–1750	11.6–27.6
		1751–2000	12.0–27.1
		2001–2250	12.6–22.0
		2251–2500	12.8–24.5
		≥ 2501	14.1–27.5

FURTHER READING

Erdemir A, Kahramaner Z, Arik B, Bilgili G, Tekin M, Genc Y. Reference ranges of kidney dimensions in term newborns: Sonographic measurements. *Pediatr Radiol.* 2014; 44:1388–1392.

Erdemir A, Kahramaner Z, Cicek E, Turkoglu E, Cosar H, Sutcuoglu S, Ozer EA. Reference ranges for sonographic renal dimensions in preterm infants. *Pediatr Radiol.* 2013; 43:1475–1484.

Haller JO, Berdon WE, Friedman AP. Increased renal cortical echogenicity: A normal finding in neonates and infants. *Radiology.* 1982; 142:173–174.

Renal pelvic diameter (fetus and neonate)

PREPARATION
None.

POSITION
Prone.

TRANSDUCER
5.0–8.0 MHz curvilinear transducer.

METHOD
The maximum pelvic diameter is measured from transverse and longitudinal images.

APPEARANCE
The central reflectivity from the renal sinus fat is less prominent than in the adult, and the cortex is iso-reflective to the normal liver. The medullary pyramids are larger and of lower reflectivity, resulting in better corticomedullary differentiation than in the adult. Normally, only a small amount of fluid is present in the renal pelvis; any dilatation of the calyces is abnormal.

MEASUREMENTS
This remains a controversial area, and each institution will have its own protocol. The following measurements are a guide.

Width and length of the renal pelvis in the fetus from 12–35 weeks of gestation		
Renal pelvis	**Male** mean ± SD (mm)	**Female** mean ± SD (mm)
Right kidney width	3.61 ± 1.1	3.51 ± 0.8
Right kidney length	4.28 ± 1.1	4.17 ± 0.95
Left kidney width	3.58 ± 1.3	3.43 ± 0.7
Left kidney length	4.31 ± 1.0	4.33 ± 0.8

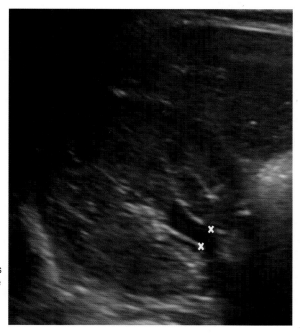

The maximum renal pelvic diameter is measured from transverse images at the point where the pelvis is at the brim of renal tissue.

The pelvic diameter measurements during antenatal imaging thought to represent groups at risk for significant renal abnormality are:

5 mm	At 15–20 weeks
8 mm	At 20–30 weeks
10 mm	> 30 weeks

Infants with antenatal renal dilatation should have an ultrasound 1 week postnatal to evaluate for severe obstruction. In infants not requiring immediate intervention or surgery for severe obstruction, repeat ultrasound and a voiding cystourethrogram is suggested at 6 weeks. If at 6 weeks the renal pelvis is < 6 mm and there is no vesico-ureteric reflux, then no further investigation is needed. If the renal pelvis is ≥ 11 mm, with caliectasis, further investigation is necessary. If the renal pelvis is between 6 and 10 mm, then serial ultrasound examinations are suggested until the renal pelvis appears normal (< 6 mm) or warrants further studies for obstruction (> 10 mm with caliectasis).

FURTHER READING

Clautice-Engle T, Anderson NG, Allan RB, Abbott GD. Diagnosis of obstructive hydronephrosis in infants. Comparison sonograms performed 6 days and 6 weeks after birth. *AJR Am J Roentgenol.* 1995; 164;963–967.

Lobo ML, Favorito LA, Abidu-Figueiredo M, Sampaio FJ. Renal pelvic diameters in human fetuses: Anatomical reference for diagnosis of fetal hydronephrosis. *Urology.* 2011; 77:452–457.

Mandell J, Blyth BR, Peters CA, Retik AB, Estroff JA, Benacerraf BR. Structural genitourinary defects detected in utero. *Radiology.* 1991; 178;193–196.

Ureterovesical jets (infants and children)

PREPARATION
Ingest water prior to the examination.

POSITION
Supine.

TRANSDUCER
5.0–7.5 MHz curvilinear transducer.

METHOD
Transverse image through the bladder base. The site of the ureteric orifice is usually lateral and defined as the uretrovesical junction at the apex of the angle between the bladder floor and the lateral wall, or in the lateral vertical wall of the bladder, above the bladder floor.

APPEARANCE
The ureteric jet is seen on gray scale when there is a difference of at least 0.01 g/ml between the specific gravity of urine coming down the ureter and the urine present in the bladder. When a spectral Doppler gate is placed onto the jet, a characteristic signal is obtained even when the jet is not seen on gray scale. Color Doppler flow imaging is more sensitive in demonstrating flow than gray scale and facilitates location of the ureteric orifice.

MEASUREMENTS
Parameters in children with normal voiding cystourethrogram and normal renal and bladder US:
- Duration of jet: Right, 2.77 ± 1.5 sec, and left 2.88 ± 1.5 sec.
- Direction of jet: Usually anteromedial and upward
- Spectral analysis: 10–80 cm/sec (mean of 31.6 cm/sec)

Frequency of jets and resultant signals increase with urine production; an almost continuous signal is obtained after a large fluid load. Although identification of ureterovesical jets may be made on ultrasound, there are no specific features regarding the jets that reliably distinguish a normal from an abnormal ureterovesical junction.

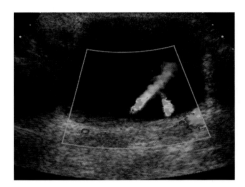

Color Doppler image of the right and left ureteric jets demonstrating the anteromedial and upward direction of the jet.

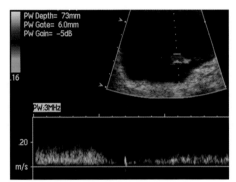

A spectral Doppler gate is placed over the ureteric jet and a spectral waveform obtained.

FURTHER READING

Cvitković Kuzmić A, Brkljacić B, Rados M, Galesić K. Doppler visualization of ureteric jets in unilateral hydronephrosis in children and adolescents. *Eur J Radiol.* 2001; 39:209–214.

Jequier S, Paltiel H, Lafortune M. Uretero-vesical jets in infants and children: Duplex and color Doppler studies. *Radiology.* 1990; 175:349–353.

12 PEDIATRIC UTERUS, OVARY, AND TESTIS

Induni Douglas, Anthony E. Swartz, Wui K. Chong, and Paul S. Sidhu

Uterus (transabdominal sonography)

PREPARATION
Full bladder prior to the examination.

POSITION
Supine position.

TRANSDUCER
3.5–6 MHz curvilinear transducer or 7–13 MHz linear transducer.

METHOD
Midsagittal section of the uterus is taken. The total uterine length (L) is measured from the top of the fundus to the external cervical os. The maximum anterior-posterior (AP) diameter or thickness is measured perpendicular to the maximum L. The maximum transverse (TRV) diameter or width is taken from a transverse section. In a midsagittal section, maximum AP diameter of the fundus and maximum AP diameter of the cervix are taken and divided to get the fundal cervical ratio.

APPEARANCE
- **Neonatal uterus:** The cervix is larger than the fundus. The endometrial lining is visible and echogenic. Some fluid can also be seen within the endometrial cavity.
- **Prepubertal uterus:** The cervix is equal to or greater in thickness than the uterine fundus, and the endometrial lining is relatively inconspicuous. The uterus presents a tubular configuration or spade shape if the anteroposterior cervix is larger than the anteroposterior fundus.
- **Pubertal uterus:** The uterine body is wider than the cervix, producing the typical adult pear-shaped uterus.

MEASUREMENT

Age	Length (L)	Thickness (AP)	Width (TRV)	Fundal–cervical ratio
Neonatal	3.5 cm	< 1.4 cm		0.5
Prepubertal	2.5–4 cm	< 1.5 cm	< 1 cm	< 1.2
Pubertal	5–8 cm	1.6–3 cm	3.5 cm	> 1.2 (2–3)

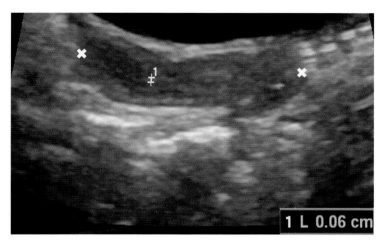

A prepubertal uterus in longitudinal length, with the endometrium measured (cursor 1). The length includes from the fundus to the external cervical os (crosses).

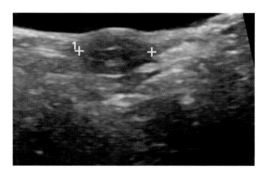

A prepubertal uterus in transverse, with a width measurement obtained (cursor 1).

The fundal–cervical ratio is a better marker for pubertal development. Uterine length shows the best correlation with age.

FURTHER READING

Garel L, Dubois J, Grignon A, Filiatrault D, VanVliet G. US of the pediatric female pelvis: A clinical perspective. *Radiographics*, 2001; 21:1393–1407.

Paltiel HJ, Phelps A. US of the pediatric female pelvis. *Radiology*. 2014; 270: 644–657.

Ziereisen F, Guissard G, Damry N, Avni EF. Sonographic imaging of the paediatric female pelvis. *Eur Radiol*. 2005; 15:1296–1309.

Ovarian volume (transabdominal sonography)

PREPARATION
Full bladder if possible.

POSITION
Supine position on a couch.

TRANSDUCER
3.5–6 MHz curvilinear transducer or 7–13 MHz linear transducer.

METHOD
The longest diameter of the ovary is obtained (d1). Maximum antero-posterior diameter (d2) is obtained perpendicular to d1. The transducer is then rotated 90 degrees and d3 is measured perpendicular to d2.

APPEARANCE
Ovoid structure between the uterus and muscular pelvic sidewall. The internal iliac vessels are posterior to the ovaries. It could be homogenous (without follicles), paucicystic (< 5 follicles), multicystic (> 6 follicles), or most frequently with multiple microcystic follicles.

MEASUREMENT

Ovarian volume = d1 × d2 × d3 × 0.523

Age (years)	Mean volume ± SD (cm³)
1	0.26 ± 0.12
2	0.38 ± 0.11
3	0.37 ± 0.11
4	0.46 ± 0.14
5	0.52 ± 0.22
6	0.65 ± 0.23
7	0.59 ± 0.25
8	0.69 ± 0.30
9	0.93 ± 0.23
10	1.15 ± 0.18
11	1.12 ± 0.43
12	1.88 ± 1.56
13	2.94 ± 1.30

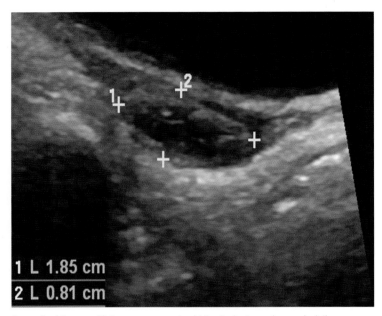

1 L 1.85 cm
2 L 0.81 cm

A prepubertal ovary with two measurements obtained prior to a volume calculation.

Mean ovarian volume is higher in girls with thelarche (onset of breast development) when compared with age-matched girls without thelarche.

The presence of thelarche is used to distinguish pubertal girls from prepubertal girls.

FURTHER READING

Herter LD, Golendziner E, Flores JA, Becker E Jr, Spritzer PM. Ovarian and uterine sonography in healthy girls between 1 and 13 years old: Correlation of findings with age and pubertal status. *AJR Am J of Roentgenol.* 2002; 178:1531–1536.

Paltiel HJ, Phelps A. US of the pediatric female pelvis. *Radiology.* 2014; 270:644–657.

Testis

PREPARATION
None.

POSITION
Supine, with scrotal support as required.

TRANSDUCER
7.0–13.0 MHz linear transducer.

METHOD
Compare reflectivity between the two sides on a single image. Obtain transverse and longitudinal images.

APPEARANCE
The testes are homogenous and of medium-level reflectivity.

MEASUREMENTS
Testis volume measurement is calculated using the following formula:

$$\text{Length} \times \text{Width} \times \text{Height} \times 0.71$$

The mean volume of neonatal testis is 0.35 ml. The mean testicular volume increases in the first 5 months from 0.27 to 0.44 ml, after which the volume decreases to 0.31 ml at 9 months, remaining stable to 6 years.

The prepubescent volume is 1–2 ml, and at puberty the volume is >4 ml.

Testicular volume greater than 2 ml allows reliable appreciation of intratesticular color Doppler flow.

There is a ×2.5 increase in testicular length and width, and ×2 increase in testicular depth between 10 and 17 years.

From the 10th year of life, the testicular volume increases ×10 from 1.36 ml to 12.83 ml in 17th year of life.

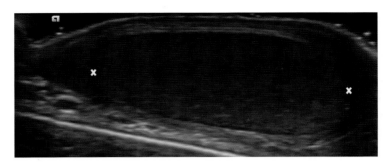

Testis volume is calculated by measuring the length (between cursors), width, and height.

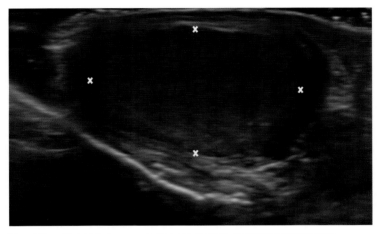

The width and height (between cursors) measurements are obtained by turning the transducer into the transverse plane.

FURTHER READING

Kuijper EAM, van Kooten J, Verbeke JIML, van Rooijen M, Lambalk CB. Ultrasonographically measured testicular volumes in 0- to 6-year-old boys. *Hum Reprod.* 2008; 23:792–796.

Osemlak P. Size of testes and epididymes in boys up to 17 years of life assessed by ultrasound method and method of external linear measurements. *Med Wieku Rozwoj.* 2011; 15:39–55.

13

NEONATAL BRAIN

Annamaria Deganello and
Paul S. Sidhu

Neonatal brain (ventricular size)

PREPARATION
None.

POSITION
Supine.

TRANSDUCER
5.0–8.0 MHz curvilinear array transducer with a small footprint. A 10 MHz linear transducer will demonstrate the superficial subdural space and superior sagittal sinus.

METHOD
Performed through the anterior fontanelle in the neonate where this remains patent. The posterior fontanelle allows access to the posterior brain structures. Oblique coronal and oblique sagittal views are obtained, and the frontal horns of the lateral ventricles are measured.

APPEARANCE
The ventricles are clearly identified as echo-free areas within the mid-level echoes of the brain parenchyma. The walls of the ventricles are well demonstrated in the premature infant but are often opposed in the term infant. Measurements are taken in the coronal direction at the level of the foramen of Monro. A minor degree of asymmetry of the ventricles is common, the left slightly larger. Serial measurements are important to document progression or regression.

MEASUREMENTS
Ventricular width: Taken from the medial wall to the floor of the ventricle at the widest point, measured at 0 mm when the ventricle appears as a thin high-reflective line; this should be described as depth rather than width.

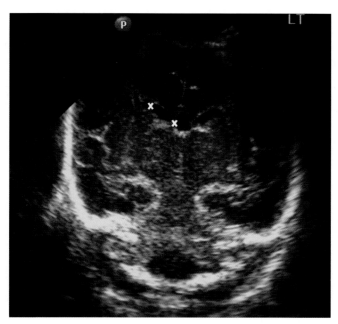

Measurements are taken in the coronal direction at the level of the foramen of Monro. Ventricular width measurement is taken from the medial wall to the floor of the ventricle at the widest point.

Gestational age (weeks)	Mean width (mm)
26–27	0.90
28–29	1.01
30–31	1.32
32–33	1.05
34–35	0.82
36–37	0.74
38–39	1.02
40–41	0.91
42	1.09

Adapted from Perry et al., 1985.

Ventricular ratio (VR): Using a transverse approach, from the temporal window (or lateral fontalle); the ventricular width (VW), from the midline to the lateral ventricle wall; and the hemispheric width (HW), from the midline to the inner skull margin, measurements were applied to calculate the VR. (VR = VW/HW).

	Term neonates mean (range)	Premature neonates mean (range)
Lateral ventricle width (VW)	1.1 cm (0.9–1.3 cm)	1.0 cm (0.5–1.3 cm)
Hemisphere width (HW)	3.9 cm (3.1–4.7 cm)	3.1 cm (2.1–4.3 cm)
Ventricular-hemisphere ratio (VW/HW)	28 cm (24–30 cm)	31 cm (24–34 cm)

Adapted from Johnson et al., 1979.

The upper limit of normal for ventricular width measured in the sagittal plane is 1.3 cm for a single ventricle and 2.5 cm for both measured together.

FURTHER READING

Brouwer MJ, deVries LS, Pistorius L, Rademaker KJ, Groenendaal F, Benders MJ. Ultrasound measurements of the lateral ventricles in neonates: Why, how and when? A systematic review. *Acta Paediatr.* 2010; 99:1298–1306.

Johnson ML, Mack LA, Rumack CM, Frost M, Rashbaum C. B-mode echoencephalography in the normal and high-risk infant. *AJR Am J Roentgenol.* 1979; 133:375–381.

Perry RN, Bowman ED, Murton LJ, Roy RN, de Crespigny LC. Ventricular size in newborn infants. *J Ultrasound Med.* 1985; 4:475–477.

Poland RL, Slovis TL, Shankaran S. Normal values for ventricular size as determined by real time sonographic techniques. *Pediat Radiol.* 1985; 15:12–14.

Neonatal brain (Doppler ultrasound)

PREPARATION
None.

POSITION
1. Through the anterior fontanelle. Sagittal and angled/ sagittal or coronal and angled/coronal views.
2. Through the temporal bone. Axial image with transducer placed 1 cm anterior and superior to tragus of the ear.

TRANSDUCER
Linear 7.5 MHz transducer.

METHOD
Resistance Index (RI) is obtained from middle cerebral (MCA), anterior cerebral (ACA), internal carotid (ICA), and posterior cerebral arteries.

APPEARANCE
The ACAs and ICAs course parallel to the image plane on transfontanellar views, providing the optimum Doppler angle. For the same reason, the MCAs are best visualized on the transtemporal view.

MEASUREMENTS

	RI
Anterior cerebral (premature)	0.5–1.0
Anterior, middle, and posterior cerebral (term)	0.6–0.8
Internal carotid (term)	0.5–0.8

Intracranial RI normally decreases with increasing gestational age.

Gestational age (weeks)	ACA PSV (cm/s)	ACA RI	MCA PSV (cm/s)	MCA RI
24–28	14 ± 4	0.75 ± 0.07	20 ± 6	0.76 ± 0.07
29–32	17 ± 5	0.78 ± 0.06	26 ± 7	0.80 ± 0.07
33–37	19 ± 4	0.78 ± 0.07	29 ± 9	0.82 ± 0.07
38–41	24 ± 6	0.80 ± 0.07	31 ± 8	0.81 ± 0.08

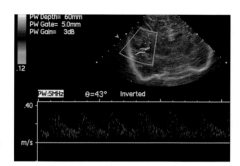

A coronal image through the anterior fontanell with a spectral Doppler waveform obtained from the middle cerebral artery from which the resistive index (RI) may be calculated.

Birth weight (g)	ACA PSV (cm/s)	ACA RI	MCA PSV (cm/s)	MCA RI
<1000	14 ± 4	0.76 ± 0.07	19 ± 6	0.77 ± 0.07
1001–1500	17 ± 4	0.78 ± 0.06	26 ± 6	0.82 ± 0.08
1501–2000	19 ± 5	0.78 ± 0.07	26 ± 8	0.80 ± 0.06
2001–2500	18 ± 4	0.76 ± 0.07	29 ± 9	0.80 ± 0.08
>2500	23 ± 6	0.80 ± 0.06	33 ± 8	0.83 ± 0.08

Adapted from Horgan et al., 1989.

Elevated or rising RI is seen in hydrocephalus and cerebral edema due to hypoxic-ischemic brain injury. Low RI is seen in babies on extracorporeal membrane oxygenation.

FURTHER READING

Horgan JG, Rumack CM, Hay T, Manco-Johnson ML, Merenstein GB, Esola C. Absolute intracranial blood-flow velocities evaluated by duplex Doppler sonography in asymptomatic preterm and term neonates. *AJR Am J Roentgeneol.* 1989;152:1059–1064.

Pezzati M, Dani C, Biadaioli R, Filippi L, Biagiotti R, Giani T, Rubaltelli FF. Early postnatal Doppler assessment of cerebral blood flow velocity in healthy preterm and term infants. *Dev Med Child Neurol.* 2002; 44:745–752.

Raju TN, Zikos E. Regional cerebral blood velocity in infants. A real-time transcranial and fontanellar pulsed Doppler study. *J Ultrasound Med.* 1987; 6:497–507.

Obstetrics

14 OBSTETRICS

Induni Douglas, Anthony E. Swartz, and Wui K. Chong

Gestational sac

PREPARATION
Empty bladder.

POSITION
Mother is in the lithotomy position. Sagittal and transverse images of the endometrial stripe are obtained.

TRANSDUCER
Transvaginal 5.0–8.0 MHz transducer.

METHOD
Average of three perpendicular diameters with the calipers placed at the inner edge of the gestational sac are obtained.

APPEARANCE
The gestational sac should be visualized by 5 weeks from the last menstrual period, with transvaginal sonography (TVS) and by 6 weeks with transabdominal sonography (TAS), as a small fluid collection with high-reflective rounded edges embedded within the endometrium, without visible contents.

MEASUREMENTS
β-hCG threshold level above which gestational sac should be seen on TVS:
- Singleton 1000 milli-international units per milliliter (mIU/mll) (FIRP)
- Twin 1556 mIU/ml
- IVF/GIFT 3372 mIU/ml

FIRP stands for First International Reference Preparation.

Mean sac diameter and estimates of gestational age	
Mean sac diameter (mm)	Mean gestational age (week + days)
2	5 + 0
3	5 + 1
4	5 + 1
5	5 + 3
6	5 + 3
7	5 + 3

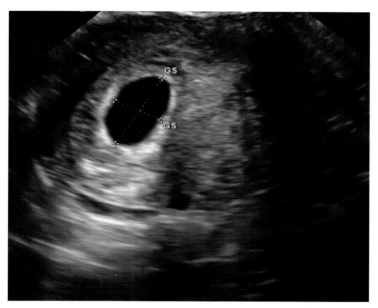

The gestational sac (GS) is measured at 17 mm in this TAS image (between cursors).

Mean sac diameter and estimates of gestational age

Mean sac diameter (mm)	Mean gestational age (week + days)
8	5 + 4
9	5 + 5
10	5 + 6
11	6 + 0
12	6 + 1
13	6 + 2
14	6 + 3
15	6 + 4
16	6 + 5
17	6 + 5

Mean sac diameter and estimates of gestational age	
Mean sac diameter (mm)	Mean gestational age (week + days)
18	6 + 6
19	7 + 0
20	7 + 1
21	7 + 2
22	7 + 3
23	7 + 4
24	7 + 5
25	7 + 5
26	7 + 6
27	8 + 0
28	8 + 1
29	8 + 2
30	8 + 3
31	8 + 3
32	8 + 4
33	8 + 5
34	8 + 6
35	9 + 0
36	9 + 1
37	9 + 1
38	9 + 2
39	9 + 3
40	9 + 4
41	9 + 4
42	9 + 5
43	9 + 6

Mean sac diameter and estimates of gestational age	
Mean sac diameter (mm)	Mean gestational age (week + days)
44	10 + 0
45	10 + 1
46	10 + 1
47	10 + 2
48	10 + 3
49	10 + 3
50	10 + 4

FURTHER READING

Daya S, Woods S, Ward S, Lappalainen R, Caco C. Early pregnancy assessment with transvaginal ultrasound scanning. *Can Med Assoc J*. 1991; 15:441–446.

Grisolia G, Milano K, Pilu G, Banzi C, David C, Gabrielli S, Rizzo N, Morandi R, Bovicelli L. Biometry of early pregnancy with transvaginal sonography. *Ultrasound Obstet Gynecol*. 1993; 3:403–411.

Embryonic/fetal heart rate (1st trimester)

PREPARATION
Empty bladder for transvaginal imaging.

POSITION
Mother is in the lithotomy position. Sagittal and transverse images of the endometrial stripe are obtained.

TRANSDUCER
Transvaginal 5.0–8.0 MHz transducer.

METHOD
Recorded by M mode or 2D video clip.

APPEARANCE
Heartbeat is initially imaged as a shutterlike pulsation at the point where the yolk sac joins the wall of the gestational sac. Usually the fetal heartbeat is observed with the embryo > 2 mm. If an embryo is > 7 mm without cardiac motion, this is suspicious for pregnancy failure.

MEASUREMENTS

Heart rate according to gestational age	
Gestational age (weeks + days)	Mean heart rate (beats per minute)
6–6.6	126
7–7.6	160
8–8.6	179
9–9.6	178
10–10.6	175
11–11.6	169
12–12.6	164
13–13.6	162
14–14.6	160

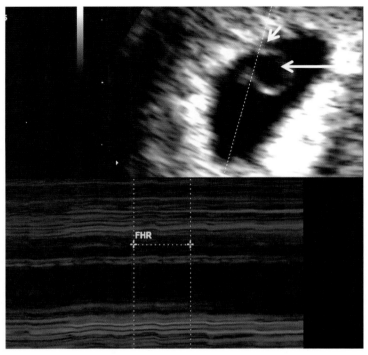

The heartbeat is measured where the yolk sac (long arrow) joins the wall of the gestational sac (short arrow). An M-mode trace demonstrates the heartbeat.

Heart rate according to crown rump length

Crown rump length (mm)	Mean heart rate (beats per minute)
1	99
2	104
3	109
4	114
5	119
6	124

Heart rate according to crown rump length	
Crown rump length (mm)	Mean heart rate (beats per minute)
7	129
8	133
9	137
10	141
11	145
12	149
13	152
14	156
15	159
16	161
17	164
18	166
19	168
20	170
21	171
22	172
23	173
24	173
25	174
26	174
27	173
28	173
29	172
30	170
31	169

Heart rate according to crown rump length	
Crown rump length (mm)	Mean heart rate (beats per minute)
32	167
33	165
34	163
35	160
36	157
37	154
38	151
39	147
40	144

FURTHER READING

Hanprasertpong T, Phupong V. First trimester embryonic/fetal heart rate in normal pregnant women. *Arch Gynecol Obstet.* 2006; 274:257–260.

Papaioannou GI, Syngelaki A, Poon LC, Ross JA, Nicolaides KH. Normal ranges of embryonic length, embryonic heart rate, gestational sac diameter and yolk sac diameter at 6–10 weeks. *Fetal Diagn Ther.* 2010; 28:4:207–219.

Crown rump length

PREPARATION

Empty bladder for transvaginal imaging. Full bladder for transabdominal imaging in 1st and 2nd trimester.

POSITION

According to the mode of scan, transabdominal or transvaginal, the mother will be in supine or lithotomy position. Midsagittal image through embryo is obtained.

TRANSDUCER

Transabdominal: 3.0–6.0 MHz curvilinear transducer.
Transvaginal: 5.0–8.0 MHz transducer.

METHOD

When < 7 weeks gestational age, the crown and rump cannot be visualized separately; therefore, the greatest length of the embryo is measured.

When > 7 weeks gestational age, the sagittal section of the embryo is taken and the longest length between the crown and rump is taken, excluding the extremities and yolk sac.

APPEARANCE

"Figure of 8" shape solid density within gestational sac.

MEASUREMENTS

Crown rump length (CRL) and estimated gestational age (GA)					
CRL (mm)	GA (wks)	CRL (mm)	GA (wks)	CRL (mm)	GA (wks)
2	5.7	12	7.4	31	10.0
3	5.9	14	7.7	33	10.2
4	6.1	16	8.0	35	10.4
5	6.2	18	8.3	37	10.6
6	6.4	20	8.6	40	10.9
7	6.6	22	8.9	43	11.2
8	6.7	24	9.1	46	11.4
9	6.9	26	9.4	49	11.7
10	7.1	28	9.6	53	12.0

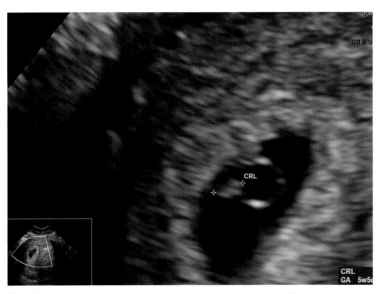

The solid density within the gestational sac is measured in the longest distance (cursors).

FURTHER READING

Hadlock FP, Shah YP, Kanon DJ, Math B, Lindsey JV. Fetal crown-rump length: Re-evaluation of relation to menstrual age (5–18 weeks) with high-resolution real-time US. *Radiology*. 1992; 182:501–505.

Discriminatory levels for diagnosis of pregnancy failure in first trimester (transvaginal ultrasonography)

PREPARATION
Empty bladder for transvaginal imaging.

POSITION
Mother is in the lithotomy position. Sagittal and transverse images of the endometrial stripe are obtained.

TRANSDUCER
Transvaginal 5.0–8.0 MHz transducer.

METHOD
Mean sac diameter (MSD), crown rump length (CRL), and fetal heartbeat are taken as described.

APPEARANCE
- **Embryo:** "Figure of 8"–shaped solid structure within the gestational sac.
- **Gestational sac:** Fluid collection with high-reflective rim embedded within the endometrium.
- **Yolk sac:** Spherical cystic structure with well-defined, high-reflective margin lying within the gestational sac.

MEASUREMENTS
Findings diagnostic of pregnancy failure
1. CRL of ≥ 7 mm and no heartbeat
2. MSD of ≥ 25 mm and no embryo
3. Absence of embryo with heartbeat ≥ 2 weeks after a scan that showed a gestational sac without a yolk sac
4. Absence of embryo with heartbeat ≥ 11 days after a scan that showed a gestational sac with a yolk sac

Findings suspicious for, but not diagnostic of, pregnancy failure
1. CRL of < 7 mm and no heartbeat
2. MSD of 16–24 mm and no embryo
3. Absence of embryo with heartbeat 7–13 days after a scan that showed a gestational sac without a yolk sac
4. Absence of embryo with heartbeat 7–10 days after a scan that showed a gestational sac with a yolk sac

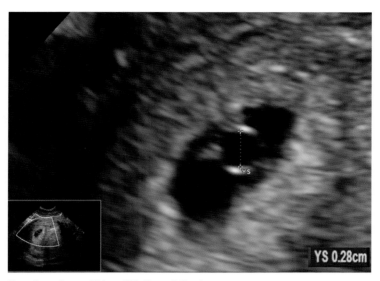

The yolk sac (cursors) lying within the gestational sac.

5. Absence of embryo ≥ 6 weeks after last menstrual period
6. Empty amnion (amnion seen adjacent to yolk sac, with no visible embryo)
7. Enlarged yolk sac (> 7 mm)
8. Small gestational sac size in relation to the size of the embryo (< 5 mm difference between MSD and CRL)

FURTHER READING

Doubilet PM, Benson CB, Bourne T, Blaivas M. Society of Radiologists in Ultrasound Multispecialty Panel on Early First Trimester Diagnosis of Miscarriage and Exclusion of a Viable Intrauterine Pregnancy. Diagnostic criteria for nonviable pregnancy early in the first trimester. *Ultrasound Quarterly.* 2014; 30:3–9.

Nuchal translucency thickness measurement

PREPARATION
Full bladder for transabdominal imaging and empty bladder for transvaginal imaging.

POSITION
According to the mode of scan, transabdominal or transvaginal, mother will be in supine or lithotomy position. Midsagittal image through embryo is obtained.

TRANSDUCER
Transabdominal 3.0–6.0 MHz transducer.
Transvaginal 5.0–8.0 MHz transducer.

METHOD
Performed at:

Gestational age (GA) between 10 weeks + 3 days to 13 weeks + 6 days

OR

Crown rump length (CRL) between 38 mm and 84 mm.

Fetus must be in the midsagittal plane. The image is magnified, so that it is filled by the fetal head, neck, and upper thorax. The fetal neck must be in the neutral position. Amnion must be seen separate from dorsal fetal skin edge. The margins of the nuchal translucency (NT) edges must be clear. Calipers must be placed on the inner borders of the nuchal line perpendicular to the long axis of the fetus at the maximum thickness. The largest of at least three good-quality measurements is taken.

APPEARANCE
Cystic area in the soft tissue posterior to the occiput.

MEASUREMENTS
Increased NT thickness for CRL is suggestive of chromosomal disorders (especially Trisomy 21), major defects of the heart and great arteries, cystic hygroma, twin-to-twin transfusion syndrome, and skeletal dysplasia.

CRL (mm)	95th percentile of NT (mm)
38	2.2
84	2.8

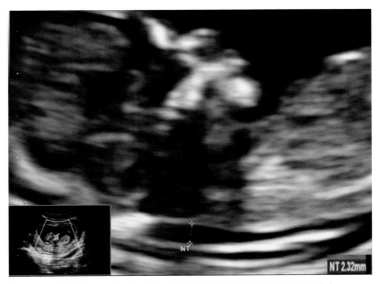

The cursors detail the position for measuring the nuchal thickness. Normal nuchal translucency increases with crown rump length and gestational age.

FURTHER READING

Ayras O, Tikkanen M, Eronen M, Paavonen J, Stefanovic V. Increased nuchal translucency and pregnancy outcome: A retrospective study of 1063 consecutive singleton pregnancies in a single referral institution. *Prenatal Diagnosis*. 2013; 33:856–862.

Hyett J, Perdu M, Sharland G, Snijders R, Nicolaides KH. Using fetal nuchal translucency to screen for major congenital cardiac defects at 10–14 weeks of gestation: Population based cohort study. *BMJ*. 1999; 318:81–85.

Pajkrt E, van Lith JMM, Mol BWJ, Bleker OP, Bilardo CM. Screening for Down's syndrome by fetal nuchal translucency measurement in a general obstetric population. *Ultrasound Obstet Gynecol*. 1998; 12:163–169.

Sheppard C, Platt LD. Nuchal translucency and first trimester risk assessment: A systematic review. *Ultrasound Quarterly*. 2007; 23:107–116.

Nuchal fold thickness measurement

PREPARATION
Full bladder for transabdominal imaging.

POSITION
Mother is in the supine position.

TRANSDUCER
Transabdominal: 3.0–5.0 MHz curvilinear transducer.

METHOD
Fetal transcerebellar plane displaying cavum septum pellucidum, atria of lateral ventricles, cerebral peduncles, and cerebellar hemispheres. Maximum distance is taken from the outer skull table to the outer skin edge. Performed between 14 and 24 weeks' gestation.

APPEARANCE
Thickening of soft tissue of the neck posterior to the occiput.

MEASUREMENTS

Gestational age (weeks)	95th percentile of NFT (mm)
16	4.2
17	4.6
18	5.0
19	5.3
20	5.6
21	5.8
22	5.8
23	5.9
24	5.9

Nuchal fold thickening has a high specificity for aneuploidy in the second trimester.

The most commonly accepted definition of "thickened" is a nuchal fold of 6 mm or greater at 15–20 weeks; however, the 95th percentile

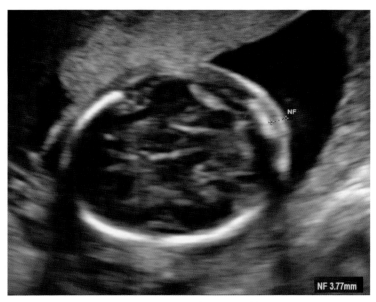

The position of measurement (between cursors) for the nuchal fold thickness.

measurement at 24 weeks also remains less than 6 mm. Thickening of the NF has greater than 99% specificity for Down syndrome.

FURTHER READING

Reddy UM, Abuhamad AZ, Levine D, Saade GR. Fetal imaging: Executive summary of a joint Eunice Kennedy Shriver National Institute of Child Health and Human Development, Society for Maternal-Fetal Medicine, American Institute of Ultrasound in Medicine, American College of Obstetricians and Gynecologists, American College of Radiology, Society for Pediatric Radiology, and Society of Radiologists in Ultrasound Fetal Imaging Workshop. *Obstet Gynecol.* 2014; 123:1070–1082.

Singh C, Biswas A. Impact of gestational age on nuchal fold thickness in the second trimester. *J Ultrasound Med.* 2014; 33:687–690.

Biparietal diameter

PREPARATION
Full bladder for transabdominal imaging in 1st and 2nd trimesters.

POSITION
Mother is in the supine position.

Transaxial image of the fetal skull at the level of thalami and cavum septum pellucidum is obtained. The transducer must be perpendicular to the parietal bones.

TRANSDUCER
Transabdominal: 3.0–6.0 MHz curvilinear transducer.

METHOD
Measured at the widest part of the image from the outer edge of the cranium nearest to the transducer to the inner edge of the cranium farthest from the transducer (as shown in image), or from the outer edge to the outer edge, perpendicular to the falx.

APPEARANCE
Thalami appear as symmetric low-reflective structures on either side of the linear midline high-reflective line (3rd ventricle). Calvaria must appear smooth and symmetric bilaterally. The cerebellum should not be present in the image.

MEASUREMENTS

Biparietal diameter (BPD) and estimated gestational age	
BPD outer to outer edge (mm)	**Median gestational age (weeks + days)**
10	9 + 1
15	10 + 5
20	12 + 1
25	13 + 3
30	14 + 5
35	16 + 1
40	17 + 3
45	18 + 6

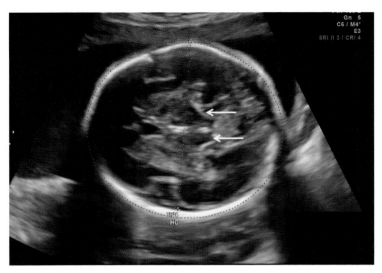

The thalami are symmetric low-reflective structures (arrows), and the widest diameter measured at this level (cursors) indicates BPD.

Biparietal diameter (BPD) and estimated gestational age	
BPD **outer to outer edge (mm)**	**Median gestational age** **(weeks + days)**
50	20 + 2
55	21 + 6
60	23 + 2
65	24 + 0
70	26 + 4
75	28 + 2
80	30 + 1
85	32 + 0
90	34 + 0
95	36 + 0
100	38 + 2
105	40 + 3
110	42 + 6

FURTHER READING

Verburg BO, Steegers EA, DeRidder M, Snijders RJ, Smith E, Hofman A, Moll HA, Jaddoe VW, Witteman JC. New charts for ultrasound dating of pregnancy and assessment of fetal growth: Longitudinal data from a population-based cohort study. *Ultrasound Obstet Gynecol.* 2008; 31:388–396.

Head circumference

PREPARATION
Full bladder for transabdominal imaging in 2nd trimester.

POSITION
Mother is in the supine position.
Transaxial image of the fetal skull at the level of thalami and cavum septum pellucidum is obtained. The transducer must be perpendicular to the parietal bones.

TRANSDUCER
Transabdominal: 3.0–5.0 MHz curvilinear transducer.

METHOD
Outer perimeter of cranium is measured. Alternatively, it can be calculated by the following formula:

$$1.57 \times ([\text{outer to outer BPD}] + [\text{outer to outer OFD}])$$

BPD = biparietal diameter; OFD = occipito frontal diameter.

APPEARANCE
Thalami appear as symmetric low-reflective structures on either side of the linear midline high-reflective line (3rd ventricle). Calvaria must appear smooth and symmetric bilaterally. The cavum septum pellucidum must be visible anteriorly and the tentorial hiatus posteriorly.

MEASUREMENTS

Head circumference (mm)	Gestational age (Mean and 95% CI in weeks)	Head circumference (mm)	Gestational age (Mean and 95% CI in weeks)
80	13.4 (12.1–14.7)	115	15.6 (14.3–16.9)
85	13.7 (12.4–15.0)	120	15.9 (14.6–17.2)
90	14.0 (12.7–15.3)	125	16.3 (15.0-17.6)
95	14.3 (13.0–15.6)	130	16.6 (15.3–17.9)
100	14.6 (13.3–15.9)	135	17.0 (15.7–18.3)
105	15.0 (13.7–16.3)	140	17.3 (16.0–18.6)
110	15.3 (14.0–16.6)	145	17.7 (16.4–19.0)

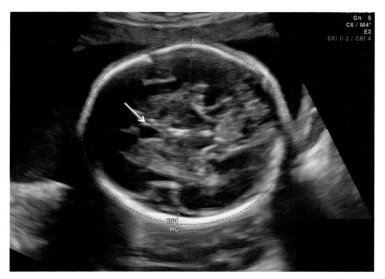

The cavum septum pellucidum (arrow) is visible anteriorly and the tentorial hiatus posteriorly to measure the head circumference.

Head circumference (mm)	Gestational age (Mean and 95% CI in weeks)	Head circumference (mm)	Gestational age (Mean and 95% CI in weeks)
150	18.1 (16.5–19.7)	205	22.5 (20.9–24.1)
155	18.4 (16.8–20.0)	210	23.0 (21.4–24.6)
160	18.8 (17.2–20.4)	215	23.4 (21.8–25.0)
165	19.2 (17.6–20.8)	220	23.9 (22.3–25.5)
170	19.6 (18.0–21.2)	225	24.4 (22.1–26.7)
175	20.0 (18.4–21.6)	230	24.9 (22.6–27.2)
180	20.4 (18.8–22.0)	235	25.4 (23.1–27.7)
185	20.8 (19.2–22.4)	240	25.9 (23.6–28.2)
190	21.2 (19.8–22.8)	245	26.4 (24.1–28.7)
195	21.6 (20.0–23.2)	250	26.9 (24.6–29.2)
200	22.1 (20.5–23.7)	255	27.5 (25.2–29.8)

Head circumference (mm)	Gestational age (Mean and 95% CI in weeks)	Head circumference (mm)	Gestational age (Mean and 95% CI in weeks)
260	28.0 (25.7–30.3)	315	34.9 (32.2–37.6)
265	28.1 (25.8–30.4)	320	35.5 (32.8–38.2)
270	29.2 (26.9–31.5)	325	36.3 (32.9–39.7)
275	29.8 (27.5–32.1)	330	37.0 (33.6–40.0)
280	30.3 (27.6–33.0)	335	37.7 (34.3–41.1)
285	31.0 (28.3–33.7)	340	38.5 (35.1–41.9)
290	31.6 (28.9–34.3)	345	39.2 (35.8–42.6)
295	32.2 (29.5–34.8)	350	40.0 (36.6–43.4)
300	32.8 (30.1–35.5)	355	40.8 (37.4–44.2)
305	33.5 (30.7–36.2)	360	41.6 (38.2–45.0)
310	34.2 (31.5–36.9)		

FURTHER READING

Hadlock FP, Deter RL, Harrist RB, Park SK. Fetal head circumference: Relation to menstrual age. *Am J Roentgenol.* 1982; 138:649–653.

Abdominal circumference

PREPARATION
Full bladder for transabdominal imaging in the 2nd trimester.

POSITION
Mother is in the supine position. Transverse image of fetal abdomen is obtained at the level of the stomach and intrahepatic umbilical vein.

PROBE
Transabdominal: 3.0–5.0 MHz curvilinear transducer.

METHOD
Length of outer perimeter of fetal abdomen.

APPEARANCE
In the correct plane, the abdomen should appear round (rather than elliptical), the ribs are symmetric, and the confluence of the right and left portal veins and the fetal stomach should be visible. The intrahepatic umbilical vein appears in short axis.

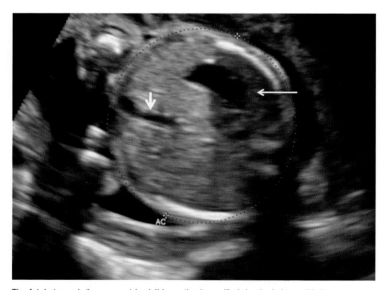

The fetal stomach (long arrow) is visible on the "round" abdominal view, with the intrahepatic vein visible in the short axis (short arrow).

MEASUREMENTS

Abdominal circumference (mm)	Gestational age (Mean and 95% CI in weeks)	Abdominal circumference (mm)	Gestational age (Mean and 95% CI in weeks)
100	15.6 (13.7–17.5)	235	27.7 (25.5–29.9)
105	16.1 (14.2–18.0)	240	28.2 (26.0–30.4)
110	16.5 (14.6–18.4)	245	28.7 (26.5–30.9)
115	16.9 (15.0–18.8)	250	29.2 (27.0–31.4)
120	17.3 (15.4–19.2)	255	29.7 (27.5–31.9)
125	17.8 (15.9–19.7)	260	30.1 (27.1–33.1)
130	18.2 (16.2–20.2)	265	30.6 (27.6–33.6)
135	18.6 (16.6–20.6)	270	31.1 (28.1–34.1)
140	19.1 (17.1–21.1)	275	31.6 (28.6–34.6)
145	19.5 (17.5–21.5)	280	32.1 (29.1–35.1)
150	20.0 (18.0–22.0)	285	32.6 (29.6–35.6)
155	20.4 (18.4–22.4)	290	33.1 (30.1–36.1)
160	20.8 (18.8–22.8)	295	33.6 (30.6–36.6)
165	21.3 (19.3–23.3)	300	34.1 (31.1–37.1)
170	21.7 (19.7–23.7)	305	34.6 (31.1–37.1)
175	22.2 (20.2–24.2)	310	35.1 (32.1–38.1)
180	22.6 (20.6–24.6)	315	35.6 (32.6–38.6)
185	23.1 (21.1–25.1)	320	36.1 (33.6–38.6)
190	23.6 (21.6–25.6)	325	36.6 (34.1–39.1)
195	24.0 (21.8–26.2)	330	37.1 (34.6–39.6)
200	24.5 (22.3–26.7)	335	37.6 (35.1–40.1)
205	24.9 (22.7–27.1)	340	38.1 (35.6–40.6)
210	25.4 (23.2–27.6)	345	38.7 (36.2–41.2)
215	25.9 (23.7–28.1)	350	39.2 (36.7–41.7)
220	26.3 (24.1–28.5)	355	39.7 (37.2–42.2)
225	26.8 (24.6–29.0)	360	40.2 (37.7–42.7)
230	27.3 (25.1–29.5)	365	40.8 (38.3–43.3)

FURTHER READING

Hadlock FP, Deter RL, Harrist RB, Park SK. Fetal abdominal circumference as a predictor of menstrual age. *Am J Roentgenol.* 1982; 139:367–370.

Fetal femur length

PREPARATION
Full bladder for transabdominal imaging in 2nd trimester.

POSITION
Mother is in the supine position. Long axis image of fetal femur.

TRANSDUCER
Transabdominal 3.0–6.0 MHz curvilinear transducer.

METHOD
The long axis of the femoral shaft is measured with the ultrasound beam perpendicular to the shaft, excluding the femoral epiphyses.

APPEARANCE
The correct position of the transducer along the femoral long axis is confirmed by identifying the femoral condylar epiphysis plus either the femoral head epiphysis or greater trochanter within the same plane.

MEASUREMENTS

Femur length (mm)	Mean value (weeks)
10	12.6
11	12.9
12	13.3
13	13.6
14	13.9
15	14.1
16	14.6
17	14.9
18	15.1
19	15.6
20	15.9
21	16.3

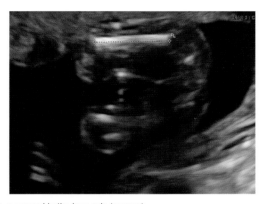

Femur length measured in the long axis (cursors).

Femur length (mm)	Mean value (weeks)
22	16.6
23	16.9
24	17.3
25	17.6
26	18.0
27	18.3
28	18.7
29	19.0
30	19.4
31	19.9
32	20.1
33	20.6
34	20.9
35	21.1
36	21.6
37	22.0

Femur length (mm)	Mean value (weeks)
38	22.4
39	22.7
40	23.1
41	23.6
42	23.9
43	24.3
44	24.7
45	25.0
46	25.4
47	25.9
48	26.1
49	26.6
50	27.0
51	27.4
52	27.9
53	28.1
54	28.6
55	29.1
56	29.6
57	29.9
58	30.3
59	30.7
60	31.1
61	31.6
62	32.0
63	32.4

Femur length (mm)	Mean value (weeks)
64	32.9
65	33.4
66	33.7
67	34.1
68	34.6
69	35.0
70	35.6
71	35.9
72	36.4
73	36.9
74	37.3
75	37.7
76	38.1
77	38.6
78	39.1
79	39.6

FURTHER READING

Jeanty P, Rodesch F, Delbeke D, Dumont JE. Estimation of gestational age from measurements of fetal long bones. *J Ultrasound Med*. 1984; 3:75–79.

Multiple fetal parameters in the assessment of gestational age

PREPARATION
Full bladder for transabdominal imaging in 2nd trimester.

TRANSDUCER
Transabdominal: 3.0–5.0 MHz curvilinear transducer.

METHOD
Simple averaging technique: Take the four estimates of age by using bi-parietal diameter (BPD), head circumference (HC), abdominal circumference (AC), and femur length (FL), then add them together, and divide by four.

Regression equations: For predicting menstrual age from any combination of these measurements (from 12–42 weeks)

$$\text{Menstrual Age in Weeks} = 10.85 + 0.060 \, (HC) \, (FL) + 0.6700 \, (BPD) + 0.1680 \, (AC)$$
$$\text{Standard Deviation} = 1.02 \text{ weeks.}$$

MEASUREMENTS

Predicted fetal measurements at specific gestational age				
Mean menstrual age (weeks)	Mean biparietal diameter (mm)	Mean head circumference (mm)	Mean abdominal circumference (mm)	Femur length (mm)
12.0	17	68	46	7
12.5	19	75	53	9
13.0	21	82	60	11
13.5	23	89	67	12
14.0	25	97	73	14
14.5	27	104	80	16
15.0	29	110	86	17

Mean menstrual age (weeks)	Mean biparietal diameter (mm)	Mean head circumference (mm)	Mean abdominal circumference (mm)	Femur length (mm)
15.5	31	117	93	19
16.0	32	124	99	20
16.5	34	131	106	22
17.0	36	138	112	24
17.5	38	144	119	25
18.0	39	151	125	27
18.5	41	158	131	28
19.0	43	164	137	30
19.5	45	170	144	31
20.0	46	177	150	33
20.5	48	183	156	34
21.0	50	189	162	35
21.5	51	195	168	37
22.0	53	201	174	38
22.5	55	207	179	40
23.0	56	213	185	41
23.5	58	219	191	42
24.0	59	224	197	44
24.5	61	230	202	45
25.0	62	235	208	46
25.5	64	241	213	47
26.0	65	246	219	49
26.5	67	251	224	50
27.0	68	256	230	51
27.5	69	261	235	52

Mean menstrual age (weeks)	Mean biparietal diameter (mm)	Mean head circumference (mm)	Mean abdominal circumference (mm)	Femur length (mm)
28.0	71	266	240	54
28.5	72	271	246	55
29.0	73	275	251	56
29.5	75	280	256	57
30.0	76	284	261	58
30.5	77	288	266	59
31.0	78	293	271	60
31.5	79	297	276	61
32.0	81	301	281	62
32.5	82	304	286	63
33.0	83	308	291	64
33.5	84	312	295	65
34.0	85	315	300	66
34.5	86	318	305	67
35.0	87	322	309	68
35.5	88	325	314	69
36.0	89	328	318	70
36.5	89	330	323	71
37.0	90	333	327	72
37.5	91	335	332	73
38.0	92	338	336	74
38.5	92	340	340	74
39.0	93	342	344	75
39.5	94	344	348	76
40.0	94	346	353	77

FURTHER READING

Hadlock FP. Sonographic estimation of fetal age and weight. *Radiol Clin North America*. 1990; 28:39–50.

Hadlock FP, Deter RL, Harrist RB, Park SK Estimated fetal age: Computer-assisted analysis of multiple fetal growth parameters. *Radiology*. 1984; 152:497–501.

Multiple fetal parameters in the assessment of fetal weight

PREPARATION
Full bladder for transabdominal imaging in 2nd trimester.

TRANSDUCER
Transabdominal: 3.0–6.0 MHz curvilinear transducer.

METHOD
Best results are obtained by using all four parameters (BPD, HC, AC, and FL), but these are not significantly different from results obtained by only three parameters. However, if using only two parameters, the combination of AC and FL will be more accurate.

Fetal weight (grams) using regression equations with two parameters (AC and FL):

$$\text{Estimated fetal weight Log10} = 1.3598 + 0.051 \,(AC) + 0.1844 \,(FL) - 0.0037 \,(AC \times FL)$$

Fetal weight (grams) using reference charts with two parameters (AC and BPD)

BPD (mm)	Abdominal circumference (mm)												
	155	160	165	170	175	180	185	190	195	200	205	210	215
31	224	234	244	255	267	279	291	304	318	332	346	362	378
32	231	241	251	263	274	286	299	312	326	340	355	371	388
33	237	248	259	270	282	294	307	321	335	349	365	381	397
34	244	255	266	278	290	302	316	329	344	359	374	391	408
35	251	262	274	285	298	311	324	338	353	368	384	401	418
36	259	270	281	294	306	319	333	347	362	378	394	411	429
37	266	278	290	302	315	328	342	357	372	388	404	422	440
38	274	286	298	310	324	337	352	366	382	398	415	432	451
39	282	294	306	319	333	347	361	376	392	409	426	444	462
40	290	303	315	328	342	356	371	386	403	419	437	455	474
41	299	311	324	338	352	366	381	397	413	430	448	467	486
42	308	320	333	347	361	376	392	408	424	442	460	479	498
43	317	330	343	357	371	387	402	419	436	453	472	491	511
44	326	339	353	367	382	397	413	430	447	465	484	504	524
45	335	349	363	377	393	408	425	442	459	478	497	517	538
46	345	359	373	386	404	420	436	454	472	490	510	530	551
47	355	369	384	399	415	431	448	466	484	503	524	544	565
48	366	380	395	410	426	443	460	478	497	517	537	558	580
49	376	391	406	422	438	455	473	491	510	530	551	572	594
50	387	402	418	434	451	468	486	505	524	544	565	587	610

BPD (mm)	155	160	165	170	175	180	185	190	195	200	205	210	215
51	399	414	430	446	463	481	499	518	538	559	580	602	625
52	410	426	442	459	476	494	513	532	552	573	595	618	641
53	422	438	455	472	489	508	527	547	567	589	611	634	657
54	435	451	468	485	503	522	541	561	582	604	627	650	674
55	447	464	481	499	517	536	556	577	598	620	643	667	691
56	461	477	495	513	532	551	571	592	614	636	660	684	709
57	474	491	509	527	547	566	587	608	630	653	677	701	727
58	488	505	524	542	562	582	603	625	647	670	695	719	745
59	502	520	539	558	578	598	619	642	664	688	713	738	764
60	517	535	554	573	594	615	636	659	682	706	731	757	784
61	532	550	570	590	610	632	654	677	700	725	750	777	804
62	547	566	586	606	627	649	672	695	719	744	770	797	824
63	563	583	603	624	645	667	690	714	738	764	790	817	845
64	580	600	620	641	663	686	709	733	758	784	811	838	867
65	597	617	638	659	682	705	728	753	778	805	832	860	889
66	614	635	656	678	701	724	748	773	799	826	853	882	911
67	632	653	675	697	720	744	769	794	820	848	876	905	935
68	651	672	694	717	740	765	790	816	842	870	898	928	958
69	670	691	714	737	761	786	811	838	865	893	922	952	983
70	689	711	734	758	782	807	833	860	888	916	946	976	1008

BPD (mm)	155	160	165	170	175	180	185	190	195	200	205	210	215
71	709	732	755	779	804	830	856	883	912	941	971	1002	1033
72	730	763	777	801	827	853	880	907	936	965	996	1027	1060
73	751	775	799	824	850	876	904	932	961	991	1022	1054	1087
74	773	797	822	847	874	901	928	957	987	1017	1049	1081	1114
75	796	820	845	871	898	925	954	983	1013	10"	1076	1109	1143
76	819	844	870	896	923	951	980	1009	1040	1072	1104	1137	1172
77	843	868	894	921	949	977	1007	1037	1068	1100	1133	1167	1202
78	868	894	920	947	975	1004	1034	1065	1096	1129	1162	1197	1232
79	893	919	946	974	1003	1032	1062	1094	1126	1159	1193	1228	1264
80	919	946	973	1002	1031	1061	1091	1123	1156	1189	1224	1259	1296
81	946	973	1001	1030	1060	1090	1121	1153	1187	1221	1256	1292	1329
82	974	1001	1030	1059	1089	1120	1152	1185	1218	1253	1288	1325	1363
83	1002	1030	1059	1089	1120	1151	1183	1217	1251	1286	1322	1359	1397
84	1032	1060	1090	1120	1151	1183	1216	1249	1284	1320	1356	1394	1433
85	1062	1091	1121	1151	1183	1216	1249	1283	1318	1355	1392	1430	1469
86	1093	1122	1153	1184	1216	1249	1283	1318	1354	1390	1428	1467	1507
87	1125	1155	1186	1218	1250	1284	1318	1353	1390	1427	1465	1505	1545
88	1157	1188	1220	1252	1285	1319	1354	1390	1427	1465	1504	1543	1584
89	1191	1222	1254	1287	1321	1356	1391	1428	1465	1503	1543	1583	1625
90	1226	1258	1290	1324	1358	1393	1429	1456	1504	1543	1583	1624	1666

BPD (mm)	155	160	165	170	175	180	185	190	195	200	205	210	215
91	1262	1294	1327	1361	1396	1432	1468	1506	1544	1584	1624	1666	1708
92	1299	1332	1365	1400	1435	1471	1508	1546	1586	1626	1667	1709	1752
93	1337	1370	1404	1439	1475	1512	1550	1588	1628	1668	1710	1753	1796
94	1376	1410	1444	1480	1516	1554	1592	1631	1671	1712	1755	1798	1842
95	1416	1450	1486	1522	1559	1597	1635	1675	1716	1758	1800	1844	1889
96	1457	1492	1528	1565	1602	1641	1680	1720	1762	1804	1847	1892	1937
97	1500	1535	1572	1609	1647	1686	1726	1767	1809	1852	1895	1940	1986
98	1544	1580	1617	1654	1693	1733	1773	1815	1857	1900	1945	1990	2037
99	1589	1625	1663	1701	1740	1781	1822	1864	1907	1951	1996	2042	2089
100	1635	1672	1710	1749	1789	1830	1871	1914	1958	2002	2048	2094	2142

Fetal weight (grams) using reference charts with two parameters (AC and BPD)

BPD (mm)						Abdominal circumference (mm)							
	220	225	230	235	240	245	250	255	260	265	270	275	280
31	395	412	431	450	470	491	513	536	559	584	610	638	666
32	405	423	441	461	481	502	525	548	572	597	624	651	680
33	415	433	452	472	493	514	537	560	585	611	638	666	693
34	425	444	463	483	504	526	549	573	598	624	652	680	710
35	436	455	475	495	517	539	562	587	612	638	666	695	725
36	447	466	486	507	529	552	575	600	626	653	681	710	740
37	458	478	498	519	542	565	589	614	640	667	696	725	756
38	470	490	510	532	554	578	602	628	654	682	711	741	772
39	482	502	523	545	568	592	616	642	669	697	727	757	789
40	494	514	536	558	581	606	631	657	684	713	743	773	806
41	506	527	549	572	595	620	645	672	700	729	759	790	828
42	519	540	562	585	609	634	660	688	716	745	776	807	841
43	532	554	576	600	624	649	676	703	732	762	793	825	859
44	545	567	590	614	639	665	692	719	749	779	810	843	877
45	559	581	605	629	654	680	708	736	765	796	828	861	896
46	573	596	620	644	670	696	724	753	783	814	846	880	915
47	588	611	635	660	686	713	741	770	801	832	865	899	934
48	602	626	650	676	702	730	758	788	819	851	884	919	954
49	617	641	666	692	719	747	776	806	837	870	903	938	975
50	633	657	683	709	736	765	794	824	856	889	923	959	996

BPD (mm)	220	225	230	235	240	245	250	255	260	265	270	275	280
51	649	674	699	726	754	783	812	843	876	909	944	980	1017
52	665	690	717	744	772	801	831	863	895	929	964	1001	1039
53	682	708	734	762	790	820	851	883	916	950	986	1023	1061
54	699	725	752	780	809	839	870	903	936	971	1007	1045	1084
55	717	743	771	799	828	859	891	924	958	993	1030	1068	1107
56	735	762	789	818	848	879	911	945	979	1015	1052	1091	1131
57	753	780	809	838	869	900	933	966	1001	1038	1075	1114	1155
58	772	800	829	858	889	921	964	989	1024	1061	1099	1139	1180
59	792	820	849	879	911	943	977	1011	1047	1085	1123	1163	1205
60		840	870	900	932	965	999	1035	1071	1109	1148	1189	1231
61	832	861	891	922	955	988	1023	1058	1095	1134	1173	1214	1257
62	853	882	913	945	977	1011	1046	1083	1120	1159	1199	1241	1284
63	874	904	935	967	1001	1035	1071	1107	1145	1185	1226	1268	1311
64	896	927	958	991	1025	1059	1096	1133	1171	1211	1253	1295	1339
65	919	950	982	1015	1049	1084	1121	1159	1198	1238	1280	1323	1368
66	942	973	1006	1039	1074	1110	1147	1185	1225	1266	1308	1352	1397
67	965	997	1030	1065	1100	1136	1174	1213	1253	1294	1337	1381	1427
68	990	1022	1056	1090	1126	1163	1201	1241	1281	1323	1367	1411	1458
69	1015	1048	1082	1117	1153	1190	1229	1269	1310	1353	1397	1442	1489
70	1040	1074	1108	1144	1181	1219	1258	1298	1340	1383	1427	1473	1521

BPD (mm)	220	225	230	235	240	245	250	255	260	265	270	275	280
71	1066	1100	1135	1171	1209	1247	1287	1328	1370	1414	1459	1505	1553
72	1093	1128	1163	1200	1238	1277	1317	1358	1401	1445	1491	1538	1586
73	1121	1156	1192	1229	1267	1307	1348	1390	1433	1478	1524	1571	1620
74	1149	1184	1221	1259	1297	1338	1379	1421	1465	1511	1557	1605	1655
75	1178	1214	1251	1289	1328	1369	1411	1454	1499	1544	1592	1640	1690
76	1207	1244	1281	1320	1360	1401	1444	1487	1533	1579	1627	1676	1727
77	1238	1275	1313	1352	1393	1434	1477	1522	1567	1614	1663	1712	1764
78	1269	1306	1345	1385	1426	1468	1512	1557	1603	1650	1699	1749	1801
79	1301	1339	1378	1418	1460	1503	1547	1592	1639	1687	1737	1787	1840
80	1333	1372	1412	1453	1495	1538	1583	1629	1676	1725	1775	1826	1879
81	1367	1406	1446	1488	1531	1575	1620	1666	1714	1763	1814	1866	1919
82	1401	1441	1482	1524	1567	1612	1657	1704	1753	1803	1854	1906	1960
83	1436	1477	1518	1561	1605	1650	1696	1744	1793	1843	1895	1948	2002
84	1473	1513	1555	1599	1643	1689	1735	1784	1833	1884	1936	1990	2045
85	1510	1551	1594	1637	1682	1728	1776	1825	1875	1926	1979	2033	2089
86	1548	1589	1633	1677	1722	1769	1817	1866	1917	1969	2022	2077	2134
87	1586	1629	1673	1717	1764	1811	1859	1909	1960	2013	2067	2122	2179
88	1626	1669	1714	1759	1806	1854	1903	1953	2005	2058	2113	2169	2226
89	1667	1711	1756	1802	1849	1897	1947	1998	2050	2104	2159	2216	2274
90	1709	1753	1799	1845	1893	1942	1992	2044	2097	2151	2207	2264	2322

BPD (mm)	220	225	230	235	240	245	250	255	260	265	270	275	280
91	1752	1797	1843	1890	1938	1988	2039	2091	2144	2199	2255	2313	2372
92	1796	1841	1888	1936	1984	2035	2086	2139	2193	2248	2305	2363	2423
93	1841	1887	1934	1982	2032	2083	2135	2188	2242	2298	2356	2414	2475
94	1887	1934	1982	2030	2080	2132	2184	2238	2293	2350	2407	2467	2527
95	1935	1982	2030	2080	2130	2182	2235	2289	2345	2402	2460	2520	2582
96	1984	2031	2080	2130	2181	2233	2287	2342	2398	2456	2515	2575	2637
97	2033	2082	2131	2181	2233	2286	2340	2396	2452	2510	2570	2631	2693
98	2085	2133	2183	2234	2286	2340	2395	2451	2508	2567	2627	2688	2751
99	2137	2186	2237	2288	2341	2395	2450	2507	2565	2624	2684	2746	2810
100	2191	2241	2292	2344	2397	2452	2507	2564	2623	2682	2743	2806	2870

Fetal weight (grams) using reference charts with two parameters (AC and BPD)

BPD (mm)	Abdominal circumference (mm)												
	285	290	295	300	305	310	315	320	325	330	335	340	345
31	696	726	759	793	828	865	903	943	985	1029	1075	1123	1173
32	710	742	774	809	844	882	921	961	1004	1048	1094	1143	1193
33	725	757	790	825	861	899	938	979	1022	1067	1114	1163	1214
34	740	773	806	841	878	916	956	998	1041	1087	1134	1183	1235
35	756	789	823	858	896	934	975	1017	1061	1107	1154	1204	1256
36	772	805	840	876	913	953	993	1036	1080	1127	1175	1226	1278
37	788	822	857	893	931	971	1012	1056	1101	1147	1196	1247	1300
38	805	839	874	911	950	990	1032	1076	1121	1168	1218	1269	1323
39	822	856	892	930	969	1009	1052	1096	1142	1190	1240	1292	1346
40	839	874	911	949	988	1029	1072	1117	1163	1212	1262	1315	1369
41	857	892	929	968	1008	1049	1093	1138	1185	1234	1285	1338	1393
42	875	911	948	987	1028	1070	1114	1159	1207	1256	1308	1361	1417
43	893	930	968	1007	1048	1091	1135	1181	1229	1279	1331	1385	1442
44	912	949	987	1027	1069	1112	1157	1204	1252	1303	1355	1410	1467
45	932	969	1008	1048	1090	1134	1179	1226	1275	1326	1380	1435	1492
46	951	989	1028	1069	1112	1156	1202	1249	1299	1351	1404	1406	1618
47	971	1010	1049	1091	1134	1178	1225	1273	1323	1375	1430	1486	1545
48	992	1031	1071	1113	1156	1201	1248	1297	1348	1401	1455	1512	1571
49	1013	1052	1093	1135	1179	1225	1272	1322	1373	1426	1482	1539	1599
50	1034	1074	1115	1158	1203	1249	1297	1347	1399	1452	1508	1566	1626

BPD (mm)	345	340	335	330	325	320	315	310	305	300	295	290	285
51	1655	1594	1535	1479	1425	1372	1322	1273	1226	1181	1138	1096	1056
52	1683	1622	1563	1506	1451	1398	1347	1298	1251	1205	1161	1119	1078
53	1713	1651	1591	1533	1478	1425	1373	1323	1276	1229	1185	1142	1101
54	1742	1680	1620	1562	1506	1452	1399	1349	1301	1254	1209	1166	1124
55	1773	1710	1649	1590	1534	1479	1426	1376	1327	1279	1234	1190	1148
56	1803	1740	1678	1619	1562	1507	1454	1402	1353	1305	1259	1215	1172
57	1835	1770	1709	1649	1591	1535	1482	1430	1380	1332	1285	1240	1197
58	1866	1802	1739	1679	1621	1564	1510	1458	1407	1358	1311	1266	1222
59	1899	1834	1770	1710	1651	1594	1539	1486	1435	1386	1338	1292	1248
60	1932	1866	1802	1741	1682	1624	1569	1515	1464	1414	1366	1319	1274
61	1965	1899	1835	1773	1713	1655	1599	1545	1493	1442	1393	1346	1301
62	1999	1932	1868	1805	1745	1686	1630	1575	1522	1471	1422	1374	1328
63	2034	1967	1901	1838	1777	1718	1661	1606	1552	1501	1451	1403	1356
64	2069	2001	1935	1872	1810	1751	1693	1637	1583	1531	1481	1432	1385
65	2105	2037	1970	1906	1844	1784	1725	1669	1615	1562	1511	1462	1414
66	2142	2073	2006	1941	1878	1817	1759	1702	1647	1594	1542	1492	1444
67	2179	2109	2042	1976	1913	1852	1792	1735	1679	1626	1574	1523	1474
68	2217	2147	2078	2012	1949	1887	1827	1769	1713	1658	1606	1555	1505
69	2255	2184	2116	2049	1985	1922	1862	1803	1747	1692	1639	1587	1537
70	2295	2223	2154	2087	2022	1959	1898	1839	1781	1726	1672	1620	1570

BPD (mm)	345	340	335	330	325	320	315	310	305	300	295	290	285
71	2334	2262	2193	2125	2059	1996	1934	1875	1817	1761	1706	1654	1603
72	2375	2302	2232	2164	2098	2044	1971	1911	1853	1796	1741	1688	1636
73	2416	2343	2272	2203	2137	2072	2009	1948	1890	1832	1777	1723	1671
74	2458	2384	2313	2244	2176	2111	2048	1987	1927	1869	1813	1759	1706
75	2501	2426	2354	2265	2217	2151	2087	2025	1965	1907	1850	1795	1742
76	2544	2469	2397	2326	2258	2192	2127	2065	2004	1945	1888	1833	1779
77	2588	2513	2440	2369	2300	2233	2168	2105	2044	1985	1927	1871	1816
78	2633	2557	2484	2412	2343	2275	2210	2146	2085	2025	1966	1910	1855
79	2679	2603	2528	2456	2386	2318	2252	2188	2126	2065	2006	1949	1894
80	2725	2649	2574	2501	2431	2362	2296	2231	2168	2107	2048	1990		1934
81	2773	2695	2620	2547	2476	2407	2340	2275	2211	2149	2089	2031	1975
82	2821	2743	2667	2594	2522	2462	2385	2319	2255	2193	2132	2073	2016
83	2870	2791	2715	2641	2569	2499	2431	2364	2300	2237	2174	2116	2059
84	2920	2841	2764	2689	2617	2546	2477	2410	2345	2282	2220	2160	2102
85	2970	2891	2814	2739	2665	2594	2525	2457	2392	2328	2266	2205	2146
86	3022	2942	2864	2789	2715	2643	2573	2505	2439	2375	2312	2251	2192
87	3074	2994	2916	2840	2765	2693	2623	2554	2488	2423	2359	2298	2238
88	3128	3047	2968	2892	2817	2744	2673	2604	2537	2472	2408	2346	2285
89	3182	3101	3021	29"	2869	2796	2725	2655	2587	2521	2457	2394	2333
90	3237	3155	3076	2998	2923	2849	2777	2707		2639	2572	2507	2444	2382

BPD (mm)	285	290	295	300	305	310	315	320	325	330	335	340	345
91	2433	2495	2559	2624	2691	2760	2830	2903	2977	3053	3131	3211	3293
92	2484	2547	2611	2677	2744	2814	2885	2958	3032	3109	3187	3268	3350
93	2536	2599	2664	2731	2799	2869	2940	3014	3089	3166	3245	3326	3409
94	2590	2653	2719	2786	2854	2925	2997	3070	3146	3224	3303	3384	3468
95	2644	2709	2774	2842	2911	2982	3054	3129	3205	3283	3362	3444	3528
96	2700	2765	2831	2899	2969	3040	3113	3188	3264	3343	3423	3505	3589
97	2757	2822	2889	2958	3028	3099	3173	3248	3325	3404	3484	3567	3651
98	2815	2881	2948	3017	3088	3160	3234	3309	3387	3466	3547	3630	3715
99	2874	2941	3009	3078	3149	3222	3296	3372	3450	3529	3611	3694	3779
100	2935	3002	3070	3140	3211	3285	3359	3436	3514	3594	3767	3759	3845

Fetal weight (grams) using reference charts with two parameters (AC and BPD)

BPD (mm)	Abdominal circumference (mm)										
	350	355	360	365	370	375	380	385	390	395	400
31	1225	1279	1336	1396	1458	1523	1591	1661	1735	1812	1893
32	1246	1301	1358	1418	1481	1546	1615	1686	1761	1838	1920
33	1267	1323	1381	1441	1504	1570	1639	1711	1786	1865	1946
34	1289	1345	1403	1464	1528	1595	1664	1737	1812	1891	1973
35	1311	1367	1426	1488	1552	1619	1689	1762	1839	1918	2001
36	1333	1390	1450	1512	1577	1645	1715	1789	1865	1945	2029
37	1356	1413	1474	1536	1602	1670	1741	1815	1893	1973	2057
38	1379	1437	1498	1561	1627	1696	1768	1842	1920	2001	2086
39	1402	1461	1523	1586	1653	1722	1794	1870	1948	2030	2115
40	1426	1486	1548	1612	1679	1749	1822	1898	1977	2059	2145
41	1451	1511	1573	1638	1706	1776	1849	1926	2005	2088	2174
42	1475	1536	1599	1664	1733	1804	1878	1954	2035	2118	2205
43	1500	1562	1625	1691	1760	1832	1906	1984	2064	2148	2236
44	1526	1588	1652	1718	1788	1860	1935	2013	2094	2179	2267
45	1552	1614	1679	1746	1816	1889	1964	2043	2125	2210	2298
46	1579	1641	1706	1774	1845	1918	1994	2073	2156	2241	2330
47	1605	1669	1734	1803	1874	1948	2024	2104	2187	2273	2363
48	1633	1697	1763	1832	1904	1976	2055	2136	2219	2306	2396
49	1661	1725	1792	1861	1934	2009	2086	2167	2251	2339	2429
50	1689	1754	1821	1891	1964	2040	2118	2200	2284	2372	2463

BPD (mm)	350	355	360	365	370	375	380	385	390	395	400
51	1718	1783	1851	1922	1995	2071	2150	2232	2317	2406	2498
52	1747	1813	1882	1953	2027	2103	2183	2266	2351	2440	2532
53	1777	1843	1913	1984	2059	2136	2216	2299	2386	2475	2568
54	1807	1874	1944	2016	2091	2169	2250	2333	2420	2510	2604
55	1838	1906	1976	2049	2124	2203	2284	2368	2456	2546	2640
56	1869	1938	2008	2082	2158	2237	2319	2403	2491	2582	2677
57	1901	1970	2041	2115	2192	2272	2354	2439	2528	2619	2714
58	1934	2003	2075	2150	2227	2307	2390	2475	2564	2657	2752
59	1966	2037	2109	2184	2262	2342	2426	2512	2602	2694	2790
60	2000	2071	2144	2219	2298	2379	2463	2550	2640	2733	2829
61	2034	2105	2179	2255	2334	2416	2500	2588	2678	2772	2869
62	2069	2140	2215	2291	2371	2453	2538	2626	2717	2811	2909
63	2104	2176	2251	2328	2408	2491	2577	2665	2757	2851	2949
64	2140	2213	2288	2366	2446	2530	2616	2705	2797	2892	2991
65	2176	2250	2326	2404	2485	2569	2656	2745	2838	2933	3032
66	2213	2287	2364	2443	2524	2609	2696	2786	2879	2975	3075
67	2251	2326	2403	2482	2564	2649	2737	2827	2921	3018	3117
68	2290	2365	2442	2522	2605	2690	2778	2869	2964	3061	3161
69	2329	2404	2482	2563	2646	2732	2821	2912	3007	3104	3205
70	2368	2444	2523	2604	2688	2774	2863	2955	3050	3149	3250

BPD (mm)	350	355	360	365	370	375	380	385	390	395	400
71	2409	2485	2564	2646	2730	2817	2907	2999	3095	3193	3295
72	2450	2527	2607	2689	2773	2861	2951	3044	3140	3239	3341
73	2491	2569	2649	2732	2817	2905	2996	3089	3186	3285	3386
74	2534	2612	2693	2776	2862	2950	3041	3135	3232	3332	3435
75	2577	2656	2737	2821	2907	2996	3088	3182	3279	3380	3483
76	2621	2700	2782	2866	2953	3042	3134	3229	3327	3428	3531
77	2666	2746	2828	2912	3000	3090	3128	3277	3376	3477	3581
78	2711	2792	2874	2959	3047	3137	3230	3326	3425	3526	3631
79	2757	2838	2921	3007	3095	3186	3279	3376	3475	3576	3681
80	2804	2886	2969	3056	3144	3235	3329	3426	3525	3627	3733
81	2852	2934	3018	3105	3194	3286	3380	3477	3577	3679	3785
82	2901	2983	3068	3155	3244	3336	3431	3529	3629	3732	3838
83	2950	3033	3118	3206	3296	3388	3483	3581	3682	3785	3891
84	3001	3084	3169	3257	3348	3441	3536	3634	3735	3839	3945
85	3052	3135	3221	3310	3401	3494	3590	3688	3790	3894	4000
86	3104	3188	3274	3363	3454	3548	3644	3743	3845	3949	4056
87	3157	3241	3328	3417	3509	3603	3700	3799	3901	4005	4113
88	3210	3295	3383	3472	3565	3659	3756	3855	3958	4063	4170
89	3265	3351	3438	3528	3621	3716	3813	3913	4015	4120	4228
90	3321	3407	3495	3585	3678	3773	3871	3971	4074	4179	4287

BPD (mm)	350	355	360	365	370	375	380	385	390	395	400
91	3377	3464	3552	3643	3736	3832	3930	4030	4133	4239	4347
92	3435	3522	3611	3702	3795	3891	3989	4090	4193	4299	4408
93	3494	3581	3670	3761	3855	3951	4050	4151	4254	4361	4469
94	3553	3641	3738	3822	3916	4013	4111	4213	4316	4423	4532
95	3614	3701	3791	3884	3978	4075	4174	4275	4379	4486	4595
96	3675	3763	3854	3946	4041	4138	4237	4339	4443	4550	4659
97	3738	3826	3917	4010	4105	4202	4302	4404	4508	4615	4724
98	3802	3890	3981	4074	4170	4267	4367	4469	4573	4680	4790
99	3866	3956	4047	4140	4236	4333	4433	4536	4640	4747	4857
100	3932	4022	4113	4207	4303	4400	4501	4603	4708	4815	4924

FURTHER READING

Shepard MJ, Richards VA, Berkowitz RL, Warsof SL, Hobbins JC. An evaluation of two equations for predicting fetal weight by ultrasound. *Am J Obstet Gynecol*. 1982; 147:47–54.

Hadlock FP. Sonographic estimation of fetal age and weight. *Radiol Clin North America*. 1990; 28:39–50.

Hadlock FP, Harrist RB, Carpenter RJ, Deter RL, Park SK. Sonographic estimation of fetal weight. The value of femur length in addition to head and abdomen measurements. *Radiology*. 1984; 150:535–540.

Fetal humerus length

PREPARATION
Full bladder for transabdominal imaging in 2nd trimester.

POSITION
Mother is in the supine position. Long axis image of fetal humerus is obtained.

TRANSDUCER
Transabdominal: 3.0–6.0 MHz curvilinear transducer.

METHOD
Length of ossified diaphysis of humerus is obtained. The cursors are placed at junction of bone and cartilage. Epiphysis should not be included.

APPEARANCE
The correct position of the transducer along the humeral long axis is confirmed by identifying both the proximal and distal epiphyses within the same plane.

MEASUREMENTS

Humerus length (mm)	Gestational age mean (weeks)
10	12.6
11	12.9
12	13.1
13	13.6
14	13.9
15	14.1
16	14.6
17	14.9
18	15.1
19	15.6
20	15.9
21	16.3

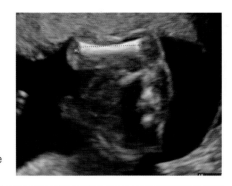

The position for measurement of the fetal humerus length (cursors).

Humerus length (mm)	Gestational age mean (weeks)
22	16.7
23	17.1
24	17.4
25	17.9
26	18.1
27	18.6
28	19.0
29	19.4
30	19.9
31	20.3
32	20.7
33	21.1
34	21.6
35	22.0
36	22.6
37	22.9
38	23.4
39	23.9

Humerus length (mm)	Gestational age mean (weeks)
40	24.3
41	24.9
42	25.3
43	25.7
44	26.1
45	26.7
46	27.1
47	27.7
48	28.1
49	28.9
50	29.3
51	29.9
52	30.3
53	30.9
54	31.4
55	32.0
56	32.6
57	33.1
58	33.6
59	34.1
60	34.9
61	35.3
62	35.9
63	36.6
64	37.1
65	37.7

Humerus length (mm)	Gestational age mean (weeks)
66	38.3
67	38.9
68	39.6
69	40.1

FURTHER READING

Jeanty P, Rodesch F, Delbeke D, Dumont JE. Estimation of gestational age from measurements of fetal long bones. *J Ultrasound Med.* 1984; 3:75–79.

Transcerebellar diameter

PREPARATION
Full bladder for transabdominal imaging in 2nd trimester.

POSITION
Mother is in the supine position.

TRANSDUCER
Transabdominal: 3.0–6.0 MHz curvilinear transducer.

METHOD
The transcerebellar plane; an oblique view through the posterior fossa that includes visualization of the midline thalamus, cerebellar hemispheres, and the cisterna magna is obtained. Calipers are kept at the outer margins of the cerebellum at its maximum width.

APPEARANCE
A dumbbell-shaped structure in the posterior fossa, behind the thalami and in front of the cisterna magna.

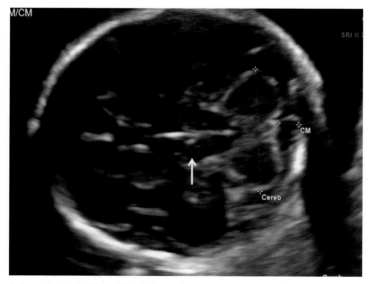

A view at the level of the midline thalamus (arrow) with cursors placed at the measuring points of the cerebellar hemispheres (Cereb) and cisterna magna (CM).

MEASUREMENTS

Transcerebellar diameter (TCD) in millimeters correlates with the gestational age up to 22–24 weeks. After 24 weeks of GA, this direct correlation no longer exists.

Mean trance cerebellar diameter according to gestational age	
Gestational age (weeks)	Mean TCD (mm)
15	14
16	16
17	17
18	18
19	19
20	20
21	21
22	23
23	24
24	26
25	27
26	28
27	30
28	31
29	33
30	35
31	38
32	39
33	40
34	41
35	42
36	43
37	45
38	48
39	52
40	55

Gestational age percentiles by transcerebellar diameter					
	Percentiles of GA (weeks)				
TCD (cm)	5th	10th	50th	90th	95th
1.2	13.3	13.6	14.5	15.6	15.9
1.3	13.9	14.2	15.1	16.2	16.5
1.4	14.6	14.9	15.7	16.8	17.1
1.5	15.2	15.5	16.4	17.4	17.7
1.6	15.9	16.1	17.0	18.1	18.4
1.7	16.5	16.8	17.7	18.7	19.0
1.8	17.2	17.4	18.3	19.4	19.7
1.9	17.8	18.1	19.0	20.1	20.4
2.0	18.4	18.7	19.7	20.8	21.1
2.1	19.1	19.4	20.3	21.5	21.8
2.2	19.7	20.0	21.0	22.2	22.5
2.3	20.3	20.7	21.7	22.9	23.2
2.4	21.0	21.3	22.3	23.6	23.9
2.5	21.6	21.9	23.0	24.3	24.6
2.6	22.2	22.5	23.7	25.0	25.4
2.7	22.8	23.2	24.3	25.7	26.1
2.8	23.4	23.8	25.0	26.4	26.8
2.9	24.0	24.4	25.6	27.1	27.5
3.0	24.6	25.0	26.3	27.7	28.2
3.1	25.2	25.6	26.9	28.4	28.9
3.2	25.8	26.2	27.5	29.1	29.5
3.3	26.3	26.8	28.1	29.7	30.2
3.4	26.9	27.3	28.7	30.4	30.8
3.5	27.4	27.9	29.3	31.0	31.5
3.6	28.0	28.4	29.9	31.6	32.1

Gestational age percentiles by transcerebellar diameter				
	Percentiles of GA (weeks)			
TCD (cm)	5th	10th	50th	90th	95th
3.7	28.5	29.0	30.4	32.2	32.7
3.8	29.0	29.5	31.0	32.8	33.3
3.9	29.5	30.0	31.5	33.3	33.8
4.0	30.0	30.5	32.0	33.8	34.4
4.1	30.5	31.0	32.5	34.3	34.9
4.2	31.0	31.5	33.0	34.8	35.3
4.3	31.4	31.9	33.4	35.3	35.8
4.4	31.9	32.4	33.9	35.7	36.2
4.5	32.3	32.8	34.3	36.1	36.6
4.6	32.7	33.2	34.7	36.4	36.9
4.7	33.1	33.6	35.0	36.8	37.2
4.8	33.5	34.0	35.4	37.0	37.5
4.9	33.9	34.3	35.7	37.3	37.8
5.0	34.3	34.7	36.0	37.5	38.0
5.1	34.6	35.0	36.2	37.7	38.1
5.2	34.9	35.3	36.5	37.8	38.2

FURTHER READING

Chavez MR, Ananth CV, Smulian JC, Yeo L, Oyelese Y, Vintzileos AM. Fetal transcerebellar diameter measurement with particular emphasis in the third trimester: A reliable predictor of gestational age. *Am J Obstet Gynecol*. 2004; 91:979–984.

Gottlieb AG, Galan HL. Nontraditional sonographic pearls in estimating gestational age. *Semin Perinatol*. 2008; 32:154–160.

Head to abdominal circumference ratio

PREPARATION
Full bladder for transabdominal imaging in 2nd trimester.

POSITION
Mother is in the supine position. Transaxial image of fetal skull at level of thalami and cavum septum pellucidum and transverse image of fetal abdomen at level of the stomach and intrahepatic umbilical vein are obtained.

TRANSDUCER
Transabdominal: 3.0–6.0 MHz curvilinear transducer.

METHOD
Outer perimeter of the cranium is divided by the outer perimeter of the fetal abdomen. An elevated head-to-abdomen circumference ratio is a sign of intrauterine growth retardation (IUGR, small for gestational age).

MEASUREMENTS

Ratio of head circumference/abdominal circumference	
Gestational age range (weeks)	Mean (range from 5th to 95th percentile)
13–14	1.23 (1.14–1.31)
15–16	1.22 (1.05–1.39)
17–18	1.18 (1.07–1.29)
19–20	1.18 (1.09–1.39
21–22	1.15 (1.06–1.25)
23–24	1.13 (1.05–1.21)
25–26	1.13 (1.04–1.22)
27–28	1.13 (1.05–1.21)
29–30	1.10 (0.99–1.21)
31–32	1.07 (0.96–1.17)
33–34	1.04 (0.96–1.1)

Ratio of head circumference/abdominal circumference	
Gestational age range (weeks)	Mean (range from 5th to 95th percentile)
35–36	1.02 (0.93–1.11)
37–38	0.98 (0.92–1.05)
39–40	0.97 (0.87–1.06)
41–42	0.96 (0.93–1.00)

FURTHER READING

Hadlock FP, Deter RL, Harrist RB, Park SK. Fetal abdominal circumference as a predictor of menstrual age. *Am J Roentgenol.* 1982; 139:367–370.

Transcerebellar diameter to abdominal circumference ratio

PREPARATION
Full bladder for transabdominal imaging in 2nd trimester.

POSITION
Mother is in the supine position. Transcerebellar plane of fetal skull at level of thalami, cerebellum, and cisterna magna, and transverse image of fetal abdomen at level of the stomach and intrahepatic umbilical vein are obtained.

TRANSDUCER
Transabdominal: 3.0–6.0 MHz curvilinear transducer.

METHOD
The transcerebellar diameter (TCD) is divided by the outer perimeter of the fetal abdomen. The elevated TCD-to-abdomen circumference (AC) ratio is a better indicator of intrauterine growth retardation (IUGR), especially in a pregnancy with uncertain dates. The TCD/AC ratio is a stable, gestational age-independent parameter that may be useful in the early detection of fetal growth abnormalities.

MEASUREMENT
$$\text{TCD/AC ratio (mean} \pm \text{SD)} = 13.69 \pm 0.94$$

The ratio remained constant throughout pregnancy irrespective to gestational age.

FURTHER READING
Meyer WJ, Gauthier DW, Goldenberg B, Santolaya J, Sipos J, Cattledge F. The fetal transverse cerebellar diameter/abdominal circumference ratio: A gestational age-independent method of assessing fetal size. *J Ultrasound Med.* 1993; 12:379–382.

Systolic/diastolic ratio in the umbilical artery

PREPARATION

Full bladder for transabdominal imaging in 2nd trimester.

POSITION

Mother is in the supine position. The spectral Doppler cursor is placed on the umbilical artery at or just before the fetal insertion of the umbilical cord.

TRANSDUCER

Transabdominal: 3.0–6.0 MHz curvilinear transducer.

METHOD

Spectral Doppler ultrasound recording of the umbilical artery is obtained:

Systolic/Diastolic Ratio = Peak Systolic Velocity/End Diastolic Velocity

APPEARANCE

A normal umbilical cord contains two arteries and one vein. The vein is larger than the arteries. A single umbilical artery is associated with fetal anomalies.

The vascular resistance of the fetal arteries decreases toward the end of the pregnancy. Early subtle increases of resistance in circulation in a compromised fetus may reflect intrauterine growth retardation (IUGR). However, the value of Doppler velocimetry in a low-risk fetus (normal weight for gestational age) has not been proven.

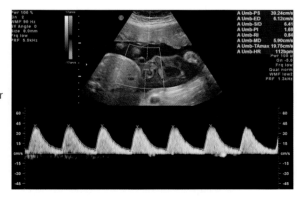

A spectral Doppler waveform of an umbilical artery, with comprehensive machine-generated measurements.

MEASUREMENTS

Gestational age (weeks)	S/D ratio (90th percentile)
16	6.07
20	5.24
24	4.75
28	3.97
30	3.80
32	3.57
34	3.41
36	3.15
38	3.10
40	2.68
41	2.55
42	3.21

FURTHER READING

Divon MY, Ferber A. Umbilical artery Doppler velocimetry—An update, *Sem Perinatol.* 2001; 25:44–47.

Fogarty P, Beattie B, Harper A, Dornan J. Continuous wave Doppler flow velocity waveforms from the umbilical artery in normal pregnancy. *J Perinat Med.* 1990; 18:51–57.

CEREBRAL VENTRICULAR MEASUREMENTS

Lateral ventricle transverse atrial measurement (atrial size)

PREPARATION
Full bladder for transabdominal imaging in 2nd trimester.

POSITION
Mother is in the supine position. A transventricular axial image of the fetus is obtained through the thalami at the level of the smooth posterior margin of the choroid plexus.

TRANSDUCER
Transabdominal: 3.0–6.0 MHz curvilinear transducer.

METHOD
Strict axial plane: The midline structures should be equidistant from the proximal and distal calvarial margins and perpendicular to the ultrasound beam.

The transverse atrial measurement is taken at the confluence of the body, occipital, and temporal horns of the lateral ventricles. The glomus of the choroid plexus is used to locate the atrium.

Calipers are placed on the inner to inner edges of the ventricle wall at its widest part, and aligned perpendicular to the long axis of the ventricle.

APPEARANCE
The choroid plexi are high-reflective structures filling the atria of the lateral ventricles.

MEASUREMENTS

Transverse atrial measurement (mm) (from 15–25 weeks' menstrual age)		
Mean	Range	Maximum
7.5	6–9	10

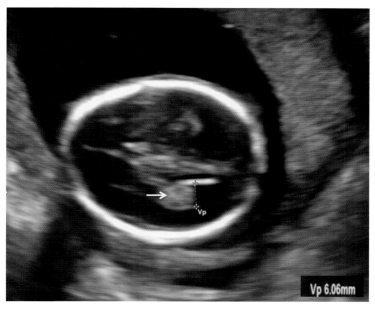

The strict axial plane demonstrates the choroid plexus (arrow) and the position to measure atrial size (Vp, between cursors).

FURTHER READING

Almog B, Gamzu R, Achiron R, Fainaru O, Zalel Y. Fetal lateral ventricular width: What should be its upper limit? A prospective cohort study and reanalysis of the current and previous data. *J Ultrasound Med.* 2003; 22:39–43.

Filly RA, Cardoza JD, Goldstein RB, Barkovich AJ. Detection of fetal central nervous system anomalies: A practical level of effort for a routine sonogram. *Radiology.* 1989; 172:403–408.

Guibaud L. Fetal cerebral ventricular measurement and ventriculomegaly: Time for procedure standardization. *Ultrasound Obstet Gynecol.* 2009; 34:127–130.

Cisterna magna measurements

PREPARATION
Full bladder for transabdominal imaging 2nd trimester.

POSITION
Mother is in the supine position. A transcerebellar view of fetus is taken.

PROBE
Transabdominal: 3.0–6.0 MHz curvilinear transducer.

METHOD
Maximum anteroposterior diameter of the cerebrospinal fluid (CSF) space between cerebellum and occiput is measured.

APPEARANCE
Fluid-filled space between cerebellum and occiput.

MEASUREMENTS

Anteroposterior depth (mm) of cisterna magna from 15–36 weeks		
Mean	**Range**	**Maximum**
5mm	2–8 mm	10 mm

Absence of the cisterna magna is suggestive of Chiari malformation.

Mega-cisterna magna (> 10 mm) is associated with chromosomal abnormalities but can be normal.

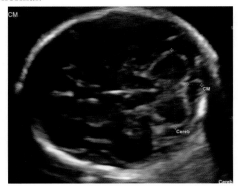

The cerebellum (Cereb, between cursors) lies anterior to the measured CSF space (CM, between cursors).

FURTHER READING

Mahony BS, Callen PW, Filly RA, Hoddick WK. The fetal cisterna magna. *Radiology.* 1984; 153:773–776.

Brown RN. Reassessment of the normal fetal cisterna magna during gestation and an alternative approach to the definition of cisterna magna dilatation. *Fetal Diag Therap.* 2013; 34:44–49.

Thoracic circumference

PREPARATION
Full bladder for transabdominal imaging in 2nd trimester.

POSITION
Mother is in the supine position. Axial image of thorax is obtained at the level of the four-chamber view of the heart with the spine in a true cross section.

TRANSDUCER
Transabdominal: 3.0–6.0 MHz curvilinear transducer.

METHOD
The thoracic circumference is obtained between the outer edge of the spine and ribs but inside the skin at the level of the four-chamber view of the heart.

APPEARANCE
Transaxial view through the thorax showing four cardiac chambers.

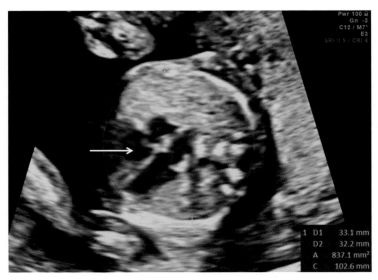

The transaxial view with four cardiac chambers (arrow) allows for an accurate thoracic circumference measurement.

MEASUREMENTS

The normal thoracic (TC) to abdominal circumference (AC) ratio is 0.89–1.0 TC/AC. A ratio of < 0.8 is associated with pulmonary hypoplasia. However, the lung area to body weight ratio is a better predictor of pulmonary hypoplasia.

FURTHER READING

Johnson A, Callan NA, Bhutani VK et al. Ultrasonic ratio of fetal thoracic to abdominal circumference: An association with fetal pulmonary hypoplasia. *Am J Obstet Gynecol.* 1987; 157:764–769.

Lessoway VA, Schulzer M, Wittmann BK, Gagnon FA, Wilson RD. Ultrasound fetal biometry charts for a North American Caucasian population. *J Clin Ultrasound.* 1998; 26:433–453.

Renal pelvis diameter

PREPARATION
Full bladder for transabdominal imaging in the 2nd trimester.

POSITION
The mother is in the supine position. Transverse image of fetal abdomen is obtained at mid-renal level.

TRANSDUCER
Transabdominal: 3.0–6.0 MHz curvilinear transducer.

METHOD
Anteroposterior of the renal pelvis diameter is measured.

APPEARANCE
Fluid-filled structure in the center of the renal sinus.

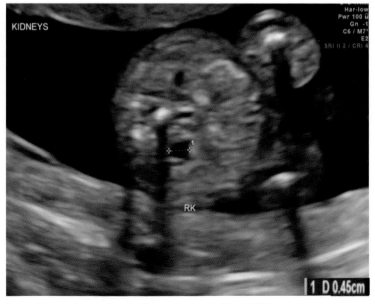

Image of the renal pelvis diameter (between cursors) of the right kidney.

MEASUREMENTS
Up to 20 weeks of gestation: < 4 mm is normal.

≥ 4 mm is suggestive of mild renal pyelectasis.

At 32 weeks of gestation. < 7 mm is normal.

Obstruction is more likely if calyceal or ureteral dilatation is also present.

FURTHER READING

Grignon A, Filion R, Filiatrault D, Robitaille P, Homsy Y, Boutin H, Leblond R. Urinary tract dilatation in utero: Classification and clinical application. *Radiology*. 1986;160:645–647.

Mandell J, Blyth RR, Peters CA, Retik AB, Estroff JA, Benacerraf BR. Structural genitourinary defects detected in utero. *Radiology*. 1991 178:193–196.

Reddy UM, Abuhamad AZ, Levine D. Fetal imaging: Executive summary of a joint Eunice Kennedy Shriver National Institute of Child Health and Human Development, Society for Maternal-Fetal Medicine, American Institute of Ultrasound in Medicine, American College of Obstetricians and Gynecologists, American College of Radiology, Society for Pediatric Radiology, and Society of Radiologists in Ultrasound, Fetal Imaging Workshop. *Obstet Gynecol*. 2014;123:070–1082.

Mean renal lengths for gestational ages

PREPARATION
Full bladder for transabdominal imaging in 2nd trimester.

POSITION
Mother is in the supine position. Longitudinal axis view of the kidneys obtained.

TRANSDUCER
Transabdominal: 3.0–5.0 MHz curvilinear transducer.

METHOD
Maximum long axis measurements are taken from the lower to the upper pole, but excluding the adrenal glands. Enlarged kidneys are associated with obstruction, multicystic dysplastic kidney, and polycystic kidney.

APPEARANCE
Elliptical structures with high-reflective margins caused by peri-renal fat.

MEASUREMENTS

Gestational age (weeks)	Mean length (mm)	95% confidence limit (mm)
18	22	16–28
19	23	15–31
20	26	18–34
21	27	21–32
22	27	20–34
23	30	22–37
24	31	19–44
25	33	25–42
26	34	24–44
27	35	27–44
28	34	26–42

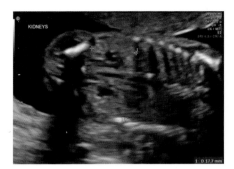

A coronal view through the kidney (between cursors).

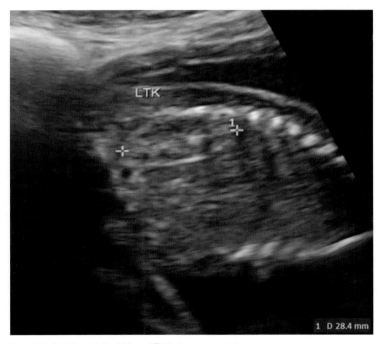

A sagittal view through the kidney (LTK, between cursors).

Gestational age (weeks)	Mean length (mm)	95% confidence limit (mm)
29	36	23–48
30	38	29–46
31	37	28–46
32	41	31–51
33	40	31–47
34	42	33–50
35	42	32–52
36	42	33–50
37	42	33–51
38	44	32–56
39	42	35–48
40	43	32–53
41	45	39–51

FURTHER READING

Cohen HL, Cooper J, Eisenberg P, Mandel FS, Gross BR, Goldman MA, Barzel E, Rawlinson KF. Normal length of fetal kidneys: Sonographic study in 397 obstetric patients. *Am J Roentgenol.* 1991; 157:545–548.

Outer orbital diameter

PREPARATION
Full bladder for transabdominal imaging in 2nd trimester.

POSITION
Mother is in the supine position. Coronal plane through skull, approximately 2 cm posterior to the glabella-alveolar line or transverse plane along the orbito-meatal line (2–3 cm below the biparietal diameter).

TRANSDUCER
Transabdominal: 3.0–6.0 MHz curvilinear transducer.

METHOD
The measurement is made from the lateral border of one orbit to the lateral border of the other orbit. This measurement may be used in place of the biparietal diameter (BPD) when BPD cannot be measured.

APPEARANCE
The orbits should be symmetric with both appearing equal and with the largest possible diameter. Abnormal orbital diameters, both hypo- and hyper-telorism, are evidence of a range of chromosomal and other developmental disorders.

MEASUREMENTS

Gestational age (weeks)	Mean outer orbital diameter (mm)
13	16
14	18
15	21
16	23
17	25
18	27
19	30
20	32
21	34
22	36
23	37
24	39

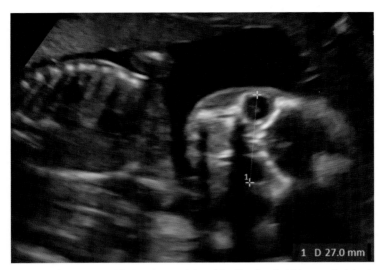

Outer orbital measurement (between cursors) from lateral border of orbit to opposite lateral border.

Gestational age (weeks)	Mean outer orbital diameter (mm)
25	41
26	43
27	44
28	46
29	47
30	49
31	50
32	51
33	52
34	53
35	54

FURTHER READING

Trout T, Budorick NE, Pretorius DH, McGahan, JP. Significance of orbital measurements in the fetus. *J Ultrasound Med*. 1994; 13:937–943.

Nasal bone length

PREPARATION
Full bladder for transabdominal imaging in 2nd trimester.

POSITION
Mother is in the supine position. Fetus is viewed in the midsagittal plane.

TRANSDUCER
Transabdominal: 3.0–6.0 MHz curvilinear transducer.

METHOD
The fetal nasal bone is identified and measured at the level of the synostosis. Care is taken to keep the angle of insonation close to 45° or 135°.

APPEARANCE
Nasal bones appear as a linear echogenic structure. Absence or hypoplasia of the nasal bone is associated with trisomy 21 and with some cases of trisomy 18 and 13.

MEASUREMENTS

Gestational age (weeks)	Mean nasal bone length (mm)
11	2.3
12	2.8
13	3.1
14	3.8
15	4.3
16	4.7
17	5.3
18	5.7
19	6.3
20	6.7
21	7.1
22	7.5
23	7.9

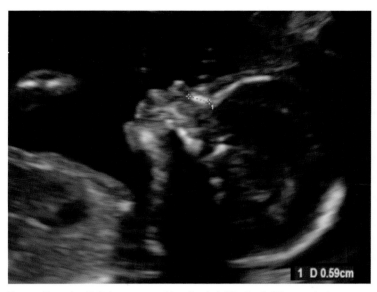

The nasal bone length (between cursors) is estimated at the level of the synostosis.

Gestational age (weeks)	Mean nasal bone length (mm)
24	8.3
25	8.5
26	8.9
27	9.2
28	9.8
29	9.8
30	10.0
31	10.4
32	10.5
33	10.8
34	10.9
35	11.0

Gestational age (weeks)	Mean nasal bone length (mm)
36	10.8
37	11.4
38	11.7
39	10.9
40	12.1

FURTHER READING

Sonek JD, McKenna D, Webb D, Croom C, Nicolaides K. Nasal bone length throughout gestation: Normal ranges based on 3537 fetal ultrasound measurements. *Ultrasound Obstet Gynecol.* 2003; 21:152–155.

Fetal stomach diameter measurements

PREPARATION
Full bladder for transabdominal imaging in 2nd trimester.

POSITION
Mother is in the supine position. Transverse and sagittal images through the fetal stomach are obtained.

TRANSDUCER
Transabdominal: 3.0–6.0 MHz curvilinear transducer.

METHOD
Maximum long axis, transverse, and anteroposterior diameters are obtained.

APPEARANCE
Normal fetal stomach appears as a fluid-filled structure on left side of the abdomen. It should be seen by 13 weeks of gestation. An enlarged stomach is associated with duodenal atresia.

MEASUREMENTS

Fetal gastric size (mean ± 2 SD) according to gestational age			
Gestational age (weeks)	Longitudinal dimension (mm)	Transverse dimension (mm)	Anteroposterior dimension (mm)
13–15	6.0 (2.5)	3.9 (2.2)	3.5 (1.9)
16–18	10.6 (4.8)	6.1 (3.4)	8.7 (6.3)
19–21	11.9 (5.5)	8.3 (5.2)	10.8 (4.9)
22–24	16.6 (9.4)	9.1 (5.0)	12.5 (7.2)
25–27	19.6 (12.4)	8.5 (4.1)	15.8 (11.2)
28–30	22.3 (15.4)	12.8 (14.4)	20.9 (13.3)
31–33	26.3 (18.5)	10.8 (6.4)	19.3 (16.9)
34–36	26.7 (16.5)	12.5 (6.9)	23.4 (16.9)
37–39	30.8 (12.4)	12.1 (2.2)	26.8 (1.9)

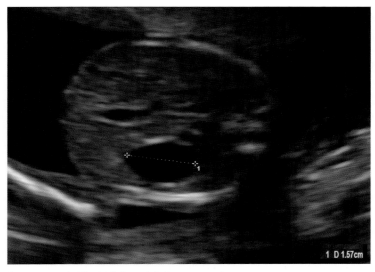

A measurement of the fetal stomach (between cursors).

FURTHER READING
Kepkep K, Tuncay YA, Goynumer G, Yetim G. Nomogram of the fetal gastric size development in normal pregnancy. *J Perinatal Med*. 2005; 33:336–339.

Fetal colon measurement

PREPARATION
Full bladder for transabdominal imaging in 2nd trimester.

POSITION
Mother is in the supine position. Sagittal view through fetal transverse colon at the maximum diameter is obtained.

TRANSDUCER
Transabdominal: 3.0–6.0 MHz curvilinear transducer.

METHOD
The colon is measured from outer-to-outer margin. A dilated colon is associated with Hirschsprung's disease, volvulus, and colonic atresia or any other distal obstruction.

APPEARANCE
The lumen of a normal colon is reliably visualized after 25 weeks with characteristic colonic haustra. An echogenic bowel that appears as bright as bone at low gain is associated with Down syndrome, cystic fibrosis, intrauterine growth retardation (IUGR), or congenital infections.

MEASUREMENTS

Fetal colon measurement (transverse diameter)		
Gestational age (Weeks)	Predicted mean value (mm)	90th percentile (mm)
26	5	9
30	8	11
35	11	15
40	16	20

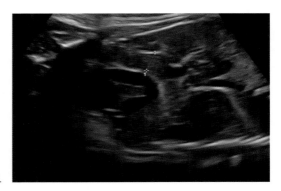

Normal colon in the
fetus (between cursors).

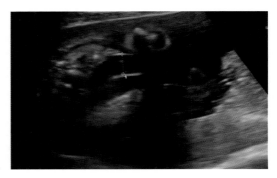

Dilated colon in the
fetus (between cursors).

FURTHER READING

Corteville JE, Gray DL, Langer JC. Bowel abnormalities in the
    fetus—Correlation of prenatal ultrasonographic findings with
    outcome. *Am J Obstet Gynecol.* 1996; 175:724–729.

Goldstein I, Lockwood C, Hobbins JC. Ultrasound assessment of
    fetal intestinal development in the evaluation of gestational age.
    Obstet Gynecol. 1987; 70:682–686.

Parulekar SG. Sonography of normal fetal bowel. *J Ultrasound Med.*
    1991; 10:211–220.

Fetal small bowel measurements

PREPARATION
Full bladder for transabdominal imaging in 2nd trimester.

POSITION
Mother is in the supine position. Short axis image of fluid-filled small bowel of the fetus.

TRANSDUCER
Transabdominal: 3.0–6.0 MHz curvilinear transducer.

METHOD
Maximum transverse diameter of fetal small bowel from outer to outer edge is taken.

A dilated small bowel is associated with volvulus; meconium ileus; and jejunal, ileal, or colonic atresia. Cystic fibrosis should be considered in all fetuses with bowel abnormalities.

APPEARANCE
The fluid-containing lumen of the small bowel is normally seen after 20 weeks. Hyperperistalsis and hyperechoic bowel are considered abnormal. (Hyperperistalsis is defined by nearly constant movement of the bowel wall during real-time scanning; hyperechoic bowel is defined as a bowel that appears as echogenic as bone).

MEASUREMENTS

Fetal small bowel measurement (transverse diameter)		
Gestational age (weeks)	Predicted mean value (mm)	90th percentile (mm)
20–25	1.4	2
25–30	1.8	3
30–35	2.9	6
35–40	3.7	8

The presence of dilated loops of bowel (> 15 mm in length and 7 mm in diameter) suggests fetal bowel obstruction.

Bowel diameter > 10 mm after 26 weeks' gestation is considered abnormally dilated.

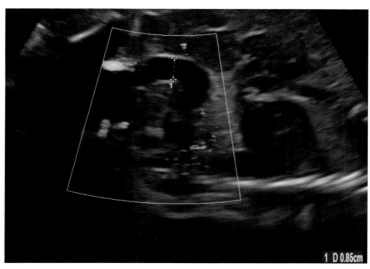

The fluid-filled small bowel is measured (between cursors).

FURTHER READING

Corteville JE, Gray DL, Langer JC. Bowel abnormalities in the fetus-correlation of prenatal ultrasonographic findings with outcome. *Am J Obstet Gynecol.* 1996; 175:724–729.

Goldstein I, Lockwood C, Hobbins JC: Ultrasound assessment of fetal intestinal development in the evaluation of gestational age. *Obstet Gynecol.* 1987; 70:682–686.

Parulekar SG. Sonography of normal fetal bowel. *J Ultrasound Med.* 1991; 10:211–220

Shawis R, Antao B. Prenatal bowel dilatation and the subsequent postnatal management. *Early Human Develop.* 2006; 82:297–303.

Amniotic fluid index

PREPARATION
Empty bladder.

POSITION
Mother is in the supine position. The uterus is divided into four quadrants using the maternal sagittal midline vertically and an arbitrary transverse line across the umbilicus.

TRANSDUCER
Transabdominal: 3.0–6.0 MHz curvilinear transducer.

METHOD
The transducer is parallel to the maternal sagittal plane, and perpendicular to the maternal coronal plane. The deepest, unobstructed clear pocket of amniotic fluid is taken from each quadrant and is measured in vertical direction.

The amniotic fluid index is sum of the maximum vertical depths of the amniotic fluid pockets in the four quadrants.

The amniotic fluid index can be used to determine the volume of amniotic fluid after 16 weeks.

APPEARANCE
The deepest pocket of amniotic fluid in each quadrant is visualized. The pocket should be free of umbilical cord and fetal extremities.

MEASUREMENTS

Amniotic fluid index (AFI) values in normal pregnancy			
	Amniotic fluid index percentile values (cm)		
Week	5th	50th	95th
16	7.9	12.1	18.5
17	8.3	12.7	19.4
18	8.7	13.3	20.2
19	9.0	13.7	20.7
20	9.3	14.1	21.2

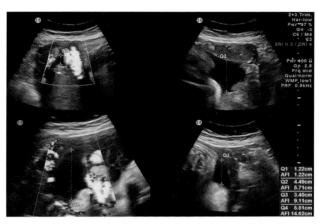

The four measurements are obtained and the amniotic fluid index calculated.

Amniotic fluid index (AFI) values in normal pregnancy		
Amniotic fluid index percentile values (cm)		
Week	5th	50th	95th
21	9.5	14.3	21.4
22	9.7	14.5	21.6
23	9.8	14.6	21.8
24	9.8	14.7	21.9
36	7.7	13.8	24.9
37	7.5	13.5	24.4
38	7.3	13.2	23.9
39	7.2	12.7	22.6
40	7.1	12.3	21.4
41	7.0	11.6	19.4
42	6.9	11.0	17.5

An AFI below the 5th percentile is suggestive of oligohydramnios, and above the 95th percentile is suggestive of polyhydramnios. Polyhydramnios is defined as an AFI > 25 cm at any gestation. Oligohydramnios is defined as an AFI < 3 cm at any gestation.

FURTHER READING

Moore TR. Clinical assessment of amniotic fluid. *Clin Obstet Gynecol.* 1997; 40:303–313.

Moore TR, Cayle JE. The amniotic fluid index in normal human pregnancy. *Am J Obstet Gynecol.* 1990; 162:1168–1173.

Nash P. Amniotic fluid index. *Neonatal Network.* 2013; 32:46–49.

Length of the cervix and cervical canal in pregnancy

PREPARATION
Empty bladder.

POSITION
Mother is in the lithotomy position. If the digital exam reveals that the cervix is already dilated more than 2 cm, ultrasound will not increase the accuracy of the prediction for preterm labor and is not indicated.

TRANSDUCER
Transvaginal 3.5–9.0 MHz transducer. (Translabial sonography is an alternative by using a 3.5–5.0 MHz transducer. However, maternal bladder should be empty.)

APPEARANCE
The sagittal section of the lower uterine segment and the end of the cervix is taken including the corner of the maternal bladder and amniotic fluid in the uterus.

The internal os, the cervical canal, and the anterior and posterior lip of the cervix at the external os should be identified.

When an adequate view of the cervix is obtained, the transducer is withdrawn about 2 cm, to avoid exaggerated lengths.

The length of the closed cervix is measured from the internal to the external os.

(At least three adequate measurements are obtained, and the shortest of the measurements is taken. During this measurement, allow a few minutes to see if a uterine contraction occurs as there can be a dramatic change in cervical length with a contraction.)

MEASUREMENTS

Period of amenorrhea	Median cervical length
< 22 weeks	40 mm
22–32 weeks	35 mm
> 32 weeks	30 mm

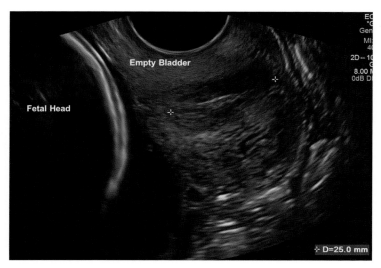

A sagittal view of the cervical canal (between cursors). (Image courtesy of Olivia Benson-Fadayo)

Between 22 and 30 weeks the 10ᵗʰ percentile for cervical length is 25 mm, and a length less than this is significantly associated with pre-term birth.

FURTHER READING

Moroz LA, Simhan HN. Rate of sonographic cervical shortening and the risk of spontaneous preterm birth. *Am J Obstet Gynecol.* 2012; 206:e1–e5.

Taylor BK. Sonographic assessment of cervical length and the risk of preterm birth. *J Obstet Gynecol Neonatal Nursing.* 2011; 40:617–631.

INDEX